Shopper's Guide
TO HEALTHY LIVING

May God bless you and your health! Kathy Jordet

For more information or to contact Kathy, go to www.
ShoppersGuidetoHealthyLiving.com or email her at
kloidolt@hotmail.comVisit www.booksurge.com or
www.amazon.com to order additional copies.

Shopper's Guide

TO HEALTHY LIVING

—Doing it God's Way—

by

Kathy Loidolt

with Dr.s John and Gail Warner, D.C.s

Dedicated to
Patty, Mike *and* **Marie Morton.**
*It is their great loss that began
many of us eating and living
as we should have all along.*

CONTENTS

ACKNOWLEDGEMENTS

Many people contributed to the making of this book. Doug and Gwen, your advice was an incredible kick start to the process. Julie, your ideas gave the book marketability. Ginger, your editing fixed my poor grammar and punctuation. Jeff, your ideas kept it grounded. Ann, you kept me inspired. Francis, you helped me remember that we are doing the right thing. Sandra and Kathy, our walks kept the book focused. John, Gail, Bill, Kristal and Scott, you taught me how to apply all of this to everyday living. Everyone at Booksurge , you worked fast and were very helpful. Matt, Chris, Stacie and Kimmy, you are my joy and reason for wanting to live a long life. You put up with my strict rules. You live out the pages of this book with Dad and me. Joe, you are the love of my life and the man who keeps me balanced. Most of all, God wrote this book and brought the right people in at the right times to publish it His way. Thank you all for taking the time and energy to help with this project. May the blessings you have given return to you "one hundredfold."

DISCLAIMER

This book is not designed to give medical advice. The federal government has declared that only medicine can cure disease. Therefore, we must advise you to seek the opinion of your doctor or health professional when making changes to your medical plan.

by Dr. William Salsman, D. C.

This is a book that every family should have. It is time for the American people to realize that when the nervous system is functioning normally and we provide the proper nutrients and avoid poisoning the body with toxic chemicals, the body can heal almost any condition. This is the one and only place a cure can come from. With all the research and money that has been spent, there is not even a cure for the common cold. Healing comes from within, not from the toxic chemicals that are found in the pharmaceuticals that so many of us are taking.

Prevention is always worth so much more than the cure. Kathy is presenting a very valuable guide to living a healthier life by teaching us to avoid the toxic chemicals that permeate our lives and by taking responsibility for our own health.

I am not a doctor, a nurse or a nutritionist and thus am not bound by any professional organization that may inhibit me from speaking out against an ingredient or product and am not required to endorse any particular method or product. I have never been diagnosed with a fatal illness and then miraculously healed myself through health food. I do not own any of the companies that make money from the items listed herein and will not be trying to sell you products. I am a wife, mother of four children and consumer health advocate who has become slightly obsessed with eating and living healthier. (Okay, my friends and family would say I have become very obsessed!)

About seven years ago, I stood by helplessly while my sister's husband was diagnosed with and later died of a cancerous brain tumor called a glioblastoma. Since then, I have watched many friends and family members receive cancer diagnoses, attended many sad funerals, and watched families try to rebuild their lives.

For seven years I immersed myself in research and natural health books to see what might help us in the fight for our health. Book after book had a constant message coming through. Whether reading a book about allergies, high blood pressure or cancer, one finds that proponents of natural health believe that illnesses common to today's society are often caused by an overload of toxins in our bodies. We are not eating and living as our bodies were designed to, and we are paying the price with our health.

It began to occur to me that it is not just my parents' generation dying of cancer; it is more often the baby boomer generation, and sometimes our children. Could there be a connection among the instant, artificial foods we are now eating, the wonderful-smelling lotions, soaps and candles we enjoy, and the amount of cancers and other diseases we are seeing? I researched, read, questioned and experimented to try to figure out what might be contributing to the apparent increase in cancers and other illnesses. What could I and others do to prevent ourselves from becoming statistics?

Conversations with friends and family invariably led people to ask me to make lists of what to buy and what not to buy. They wanted someone to take them shopping and show them what they should purchase. They wanted to be healthy, but they didn't want to spend years doing the research and reading detailed books that told them how to be healthier. So here is a quick read on eating and living well while preventing the illnesses of modern society. It is a synopsis of hundreds of health books. The ideas presented in this book tend to be universally understood in the homeopathic world. If I have read a piece of information only once or twice, it is not included it in this book. Only information that I have read five or seven, and often twenty to thirty times, is included. This information was gathered from natural doctors, nutritionists, cancer survivors, doctors of chiropractic, medical doctors and thousands of conversations from those living the concepts in these pages. Doctors John and Gail Warner have been gracious and patient enough to work through the data with me to ensure its accuracy.

If you have diabetes, attention deficit hyperactivity disorder (ADHD), depression, high cholesterol, high blood pressure, arthritis, constipation, irritable bowel syndrome, cancer, or are overweight or tired, you can change your life by eating the way we were meant to eat. However, because the FDA (Food and Drug Administration) has a law stating that only medicine can cure disease, I cannot and do not claim that the natural methods contained herein are able to cure disease, and must advise you to seek professional advice where your health is concerned. I can tell you that my family and some friends live out the phases in this book and have seen our energy, moods and athletic abilities improve, our sick days decline significantly, our weight loss become easy, and even our wrinkles decrease and fingernails get stronger.

This book includes tear-out shopping lists of what to purchase and what to eliminate on your shopping trips, name brands my family has enjoyed and references for further reading. I have included five phases to move you gradually toward healthier living. You can do these phases one step at a time, pick and choose and bounce around, or do them all at once. The time frame for each phase is up to you and your family. You may zip through one phase and spend months on another phase. It all depends on your motivation and the individual needs and likes of your family. With each phase you will feel so much better; your mood, skin, outlook and feeling of control over your life will improve dramatically.

Here's to your health!

CHAPTER 1

Different, But Still Good

The amount of nutrition information available today is overwhelming and contradictory. Eat a low carbohydrate diet; eat good fats. Eat fish; don't eat fish because it has mercury. Use sunscreen; don't use sunscreen. Make sure there is fluoride in your water; fluoride is poison. Red meat is good for you; red meat is bad for you. Poultry is good for you; poultry has hormones. Got milk? Milk causes allergies. What do we do with all of the information? How do we sort through all of the data without becoming obsessive about it?

As my friend Ann Miller says, "You almost have to become obsessive about eating healthy because no one is looking out for the consumer!" She's right, so I have become obsessed for you! Food manufacturers and producers of soaps, lotions and make-up are not looking out for our health. Our health is our responsibility. Manufacturers are interested in making a profit for themselves and their stockholders. That is the job of a corporation, to make a profit. Product loyalty is the primary tool for meeting this objective. If the consumer gets diabetes, cancer, arthritis, allergies or becomes obese because of these products, who's to blame? There is no way to trace the cancer or weight problem back to one specific product because virtually all products we Americans like to eat, smell or purchase contain some type of poison. We like things that smell good, taste good and feel comfortable. The ingredients that make things smell, taste and feel good have been discovered to be the causes of the above illnesses and many more.

Even though this is the first decade that the average American's life expectancy is predicted to decline, we still live to be approximately 77.9 years old.[1] The consumer is told by manufacturers that you have to ingest "huge" amounts of diet pop or consume "vast" quantities of mercury or other toxic metals to get cancer from them. During this seventy-seven plus years that we are on this earth, virtually everything we ingest, breathe and drink from our modern diet adds "just a little" poison to our systems. Just a little poison here and just a little poison there, three meals a day, times seventy-seven years adds up to the "huge" and "vast" quantities of poison in our systems. Our bodies are full to the brim and are not going to take it anymore! Our organs are screaming for attention. Arthritis, allergies, high blood pressure, obesity, high cholesterol and constant tiredness are ways our bodies communicate "I'm overloaded! Stop poisoning me and start eating and consuming things that help me function better!"

Eating, like many other areas in life, is best done according to God's instructions. God is the designer and maker of humans. He created us, and He left us the written Word to tell us how to do many things, like how to be a good spouse and friend, how to handle finances, how to run a church and which foods to eat. I believe that when God tells us to eat certain foods, we can "take that to the bank." If God said it, you should eat it. This book goes back to the basics of how we were instructed to eat.

God has sprinkled food words and direct instructions throughout the Bible that tell us what is meant to go into our bodies. Thousands of years later, scientists and health professionals are agreeing with many of God's statements. For instance, Leviticus 11:9 states, *"Of all the creatures living in the water of the seas and the streams, you may eat any that have fins and scales."* Cold-water fish with fins and scales are the healthiest forms of omega-3 oils and are incredible for our skin, moods and organs. Jesus ate fish several times a week and told us to be like Him (Romans 8:29: *"For those He foreknew He also predestined to be conformed to the likeness of His Son."*). Bottom-feeding fish without fins and scales and hard-shelled ocean life, like crab, lobster and shrimp have been discovered to have high levels of mercury, one of the deadliest metals to consume. God tells us, in Leviticus 11:10, that we are to detest the creatures in the streams and lakes that do not have fins and scales: *"But all creatures in the seas or streams that do not have fins and scales—whether among the swarming things or among all the other living creatures in the water—you are to detest."*

Another example is in Isaiah 32:20. God tells us, *"How blessed you will be, sowing your seed by every stream, and letting your cattle and donkeys range free."* How amazing is that! We now know that free-range cattle are healthier and get fewer diseases than stockyard cattle because, among other things, they get exercise and don't need antibiotics nearly as often.

Proverbs 31 talks about the virtues of a woman of noble character. In verse 13, she is highly regarded because she *"selects wool and flax and works with eager hands."* Flax oil and flax seed have been determined by modern science to help cure high cholesterol, high blood pressure, depression, anxiety, wrinkles and cancer. Flax oil is one of the healthiest foods you can put into your body. You cannot pick up a book about eating healthy without reading about adding flax to your diet. I have been taking flax seed and flax seed oil for seven years and have noticed that I now have fewer wrinkles than I did a few years ago.

Olive oil is talked about throughout God's word. In the Bible it is used to keep lamps burning, heal the sick and anoint the blessed (Matthew 25:1-13, Isaiah 1:1, Samuel 10:1, Exodus 29:7). Olive oil is known today to keep your digestive tract working, increase antioxidants, reduce wrinkles, lower high blood pressure, and reduce your chances of contracting cancer. [2] It can be used as a lotion to heal dry and peeling or cracking skin. (We used it on my daughter's cracking heels, and they were cleared up and soft in two days.)

The processed, packaged, partially hydrogenated and color-dyed foods we purchase at the average grocery stores are edible, but so is this paper I have written on. The paper I am writing on and anything highly processed or partially hydrogenated have almost no nutrition and are difficult for our bodies to process and filter out. The natural foods God created and identified are what our bodies need to function well. We need the sugars from fruit, the vitamins from vegetables and the oils and proteins from meat and fish for our bodies to function properly.

In 1906, America passed a law called the Pure Food and Drug Act, which was "an Act for preventing the manufacture, sale, or transportation of adulterated or misbranded or poisonous or deleterious foods, drugs, medicines and liquors, and for regulating traffic herein, and for other purposes." [3] It prevented manufacturers from attempting to pass off anything as food that was not food (and likewise for drugs and medicine). For example, it was illegal to sell white flour and white sugar as we know them today because they had been bleached. Bleach, a poison, was not allowed to be sold as a food. Only pure food could be sold for human consumption.

In 1938, lobbyists for the manufacturers of food products pressured Congress to abolish the Pure Food Act and the FDA's (Food and Drug Administration) role was expanded under Franklin D. Roosevelt's administration. The FDA allowed manufacturers to add bleach and other nonfood items to food products and began focusing on monitoring the identification of drugs rather than the purity of foods.[4] The institution of the FDA allowed food manufacturers to sell bleached, refined flour and sugar to the unsuspecting public. As you can imagine, this new flour was softer, prettier and much cleaner looking than its pure food counterpart.

The very organization that we rely on to protect us allows poisons, like bleach, to be added to our food so the products will taste better and look better and encourage us to purchase more of them. It has been going on for so long that the average consumer cannot distinguish the poison from the food they should be eating. We think Fruit Roll-Ups have fruit in them; so they are good for our kids, right? Juice and milk are pasteurized to prevent the consumer from getting sick, yet pasteurizing heats juice and kills off all enzymes and vitamins, leaving a sugary drink that lowers our immune system. As a population, we have begun to get cancers and are unable to identify which products have contributed to our illnesses. Virtually everything we eat, drink, wash with and rub on our bodies has contributed to it. The makers of these products are off the hook, and we are left trying to figure out what went wrong with our health.

High fructose corn syrup (HFCS) is a by-product of corn and may contain many times the fructose (a form of sugar) that sugar contains. The corn used to produce high fructose corn syrup is often genetically modified. It is much cheaper to produce than regular sugar and and may cause you to crave more. All sugars inhibit the white blood cells in your body and change the collagen in your skin, which in turn increases wrinkles and aging. It can inhibit the absorption of copper, which may lead to bone fragility, anemia and defects of the connective tissues, arteries and bones. It has been connected to infertility, heart arrhythmias, high cholesterol, heart attacks and diabetes. [5]

When Linda Joyce Forristal, with the Weston A. Price Foundation, conducted experiments with rats, she found that high fructose corn syrup caused the rats' livers to look like those of alcoholics'. One cannot help but wonder: if HFCS is a concentrated form of sugar and the pancreas' job is to process sugar, could there be a connection between the increased use of HFCS and pancreatic cancer? You will find high fructose corn syrup in almost all sweet foods that you enjoy, including soda pop, candy, juices, fruit snacks and even breads. The Standard American Diet (SAD) is so full of processed, refined and highly flavored foods like HFCS that we have no appetite for the real food, designed by God, that our bodies need.

We were created with absolutely incredible filtering systems. The liver, kidneys, gallbladder, lymph system and skin are all capable of detoxifying and processing out vast amounts of poison, foreign particles and waste products. Until recent generations, these filtering organs could generally keep up with the poisons the average individual consumed. However, with the onslaught of preserved, color-dyed and hormone-laced foods we eat, along with the modern lotions, shampoos and soaps we put on our skin, and the chemicals we breathe, drink and take daily, we Americans have found the saturation point of these incredible filtering systems.

Each time we pop a chemically produced prescription pill or choose processed food over food from nature, we are adding to the strain on our filtering systems. Our overloaded organs send the excess poisons they cannot filter back into our bloodstreams. These poisons may settle into the weakest parts of our bodies, modifying cells and causing disorders.

For some it becomes asthma; for others allergies, diabetes, high blood pressure, high cholesterol, depression, cancer, arthritis, etc.

Adding more prescription pills to cover the symptoms of our modern lifestyle will only add to the problems our filtering systems are dealing with. Does it worry you that prescription medications come with half-page disclaimers about the side effects they may cause, "including death"? These drugs are not food but are foreign objects that are not meant to be in our bodies. They are adding to the strain on our internal filtering system. As Lorraine Day, M.D., an alternative therapy proponent, reminds us, "If you have a headache, your body does not have a shortage of Tylenol. When you have cancer, your body does not have a shortage of chemotherapy."[6]

We as individuals have to choose to find healthy foods that taste as my sister, Patty, puts it, "different, but still good." Healthy food does not have the incredible-tasting, addictive flavors that commercial foods have. It does take time to get used to the new tastes. Your kids will tell you "it's gross" because their taste buds have been desensitized by our Standard American Diet. I remind my children this food will be different, but that they don't have a choice. I tell them I will not intentionally "poison" them anymore. Eventually, they get used to the tastes. After eating food in its natural form, the way it was meant to be eaten, our taste buds adjust, and we don't need to have the sugars and flavor additives of our modern society as often. It has become okay to eat differently than our society does. Our family chooses to eat by the Bible, just as our family tries to live by the Bible. We have found that the Veggie Tales videos are right: "God's way is not always the easy way, but it is always the best way"[7]

We still crave the high-sugar foods on occasion. About once a month (more often at first), we celebrate how well we are eating by getting what we crave because, as my husband put it, "Let's not kid ourselves, that stuff tastes good."

I was a sugar-holic before my brother-in-law, Lee, died of brain cancer. When I fasted from chocolate, I didn't eat anything because virtually everything I ate contained chocolate (and therefore sugar). There were many nights in earlier years that my dinner consisted of a box of cookies. After Lee was diagnosed, my sister investigated possible causes of cancer and began teaching us about some of the theories in this book. If a sugar-holic like me can go from having chocolate at almost every meal to eating God's way and actually craving healthy meals, anyone can do it! Before changing our diets, my family used to go to fast-food restaurants at least once a week. No more! And we feel better because of the change. We have a very picky eater at our house. If she can do this diet, any child can. You and your family can too! Really!

CHAPTER 2

Phase I
The Easy Changes

I n Phase One, you begin by making the easy changes: swapping one purchase for another seemingly more expensive, yet healthier item. Initially, you will spend more on your groceries and personal items. Whole Foods will provide large selections and great produce. With this large selection, they have both organic and non-organic produce and a few non-organic stock items – just check labels. The Natural Grocer/Vitamin Cottage stores thoroughly check products before they go on the shelf. Get to know your local store and their policies.

After you have shopped the local health food stores for a while and have found brands your family likes, you will be able to switch over to Internet purchasing and bulk buying for dry goods and co-op sales for perishables. See the resources section for retailers that provide this service. Costco also has organic fruit, and most mainstream grocery stores are beginning to carry organic produce and other items. I usually find their selection and quality to be limited but use them when needed. After purchasing organic products for two years, I compared my current monthly grocery bill to a grocery bill a few years earlier and found a difference of about 10 percent per month. However, this difference is partially offset by a decrease in doctor visits, zero spent on prescription drugs, and a reduction in restaurant and convenience food bills. It is well worth the changes I have seen in the health of my family.

If your family is struggling to get started, allow each person to "choose their poison". Pick 1-3 things that they do not want to give up just yet, the food items that are too important for them right now. Allow each person to continue eating these chosen poisons until they are used to the program and see the rewards of this new lifestyle. We'll have more success if we don't have to give up everything right away.

In Phase I, you will begin by purchasing or using the following items:

> Extra virgin olive oil—first cold-pressed
> Walnut oil
> Free range eggs with omega-3
> Organic butter
> Organic fruits and vegetables
> Sprouted Grain breads/Great Harvest/Rudy's
> > Organic Bread
> POM juice
> Flax seed
> Hormone-free red meat
> Hormone-free chicken
> Natural chips
> Organic crackers and cookies
> Natural ice cream

In Phase I, you will eliminate or avoid the following items:

> Partially hydrogenated oils
> High fructose corn syrup
> Vegetable/canola oils
> Lard and Crisco
> Margarine
> White bread
> Non-organic fruits/vegetables
> Clothes dryer sheets
> Red meat with hormones
> Chicken with hormones
> Non organic crackers and chips
> Most ice creams

Extra virgin olive oil (EVOO) can and should replace all your other vegetable oils. I did it across the board in pancakes, recipes, meat dishes and lightly fried foods. No one at my house complained, although I expected them to notice. If you have a family with sensitive taste buds, start with the light version and phase over to regular extra virgin olive oil. Look for metal cans or bottles with the dark glass containers as it keeps the light from breaking down the oil and helps it last longer. Buy "first press cold-processed" olive oil. Heat processing oil at manufacturing plants, as is done with other vegetable and corn oils, chemically alters the oil and causes free radicals to be released. Consuming these altered oils will cause free radical damage to your cells, increasing your chances of cancer.

A free radical is an unstable, toxic molecule of oxygen that is missing an electron. It destroys healthy molecules. The process develops when molecules within cells react with oxygen, or oxidize. Free radicals then begin to break down cells, especially the cell membranes, and harmfully alter proteins, enzymes and even

DNA. Sources of free radicals include pesticides, industrial pollutants and tobacco smoke.[8] Uncontrolled free radical production plays a major role in the development of degenerative diseases including cancer, heart disease, atherosclerosis, Alzheimer's, cataracts, osteoarthritis, immune deficiencies and aging. Free radical damage can be reduced by consuming omega-3 oils.

Walnut Oil is also a cold-processed oil. It can withstand higher temperatures than olive oil when used for cooking. At home, we use walnut oil for frying at moderate temperatures. Frying at high temperatures is not as healthy for you because, whether oil is heated to high temperatures at home or in a processing plant, high temperatures chemically alter the makeup of the cells in the oil. Ingesting these altered oils can cause free radical damage in our bodies. At my house, we try to cook food at the lowest temperature we can. It is still nice to have walnut oil around for some of your cooking. The milder taste makes it great for use in recipes.

Free-range chickens are chickens that are allowed to run around free, rather than being locked up in a cage. They produce free-range eggs. The shells from free-range eggs are thicker because, like us, chickens are healthier when they can get some exercise. Free range practices make stronger bones, muscles and eggs for the chicken—and for us. It is even more of a plus if the chickens are fed omega-3 seeds and oils.

Organic butter is produced from cows that were not given growth hormones or antibiotics and were not fed the body parts of dead animals (explained shortly).

Organic fruits and vegetables are produced without pesticides. Pesticides are poison. They kill bugs; and if we eat enough of them, they will do the same to us. You still need to wash organic produce with water or a vegetable wash to prevent ingestion of microscopic organisms and germs.

I am often asked what the term "organic" means. The Organic Foods Production Act (OFPA) of 1990 required the USDA (United States Department of Agriculture) to develop national organic standards for organically produced agriculture. The final regulations for implementation of the OFPA were published in the Federal Register in December 2000. The new rule took effect April 21, 2001; full compliance was required by October 20, 2002. Among other things, organic certification meant that a farmer must have an organic farm plan, maintain a paper trail for materials applied, and undergo an annual farm inspection by an accredited certification organization.

Organic food is produced by farmers who emphasize the use of renewable resources and the conservation of soil and water to enhance environmental quality for future generations. Organic meat, poultry, eggs and dairy products come from animals that are given no antibiotics or growth hormones. Organic food is produced without using most conventional pesticides, petroleum-based or sewage-based fertilizers, bioengineering or ionizing radiation. Before a product can be labeled "organic," a government-approved certifier inspects the farm where food is grown to make sure the farmer is following all rules necessary to meet USDA organic standards. Companies that handle or process organic food before it gets to your local supermarket or restaurant must also be certified. [9]

Ezekiel Sprouted Grain Bread is produced from the sprouted form of different grains and lentils listed in Ezekiel 4:9: *"Take wheat and barley, beans and lentils, millet and spelt; put them in a storage jar and use them to make bread for yourself. "* Not only does our creator directly tell us to eat these things together, but modern science has agreed that the sprouted form of any food is the healthiest way to eat that food. The sprouted form of a plant is packed with nutrients that the plant needs to grow. Ezekiel

Bread is probably drier than the breads you are used to. My kids like it for sandwiches but not toast. If your family is not happy with Ezekiel Bread, you may try breads from Great Harvest or Rudy's Organic Breads. They do not contain color dyes or high fructose corn syrup and are closer to tastes we are used to. Later you may be able to phase your kids over to the Ezekiel Breads.

POM Juice is a brand of pomegranate juice. It is a cold-processed juice. When a juice is pasteurized, the manufacturer must heat the juice. Heating the juice also kills off all the enzymes the fruit contained. These enzymes were designed by God to help our bodies digest the fruit and/or juice. Heat processing also takes out the vitamins and minerals that the fruit used to contain and leaves only the sugars. Cold-processed juices are hard to come by, but provide our bodies with enzymes, vitamins and minerals that we need.

Pomegranates are written about in the Song of Songs. The juice is full of antioxidants and tastes wonderful. At home, we use it as our new treat. You will only find this juice in the refrigerator section and need to keep it refrigerated. We prefer the blueberry POM juice to other organic juices.

Flax seed is full of omega-3 oils that combat the damage caused by free radicals. It helps reduce cholesterol, high blood pressure, anxiety, depression, wrinkles associated with aging, cancer, arthritis and many more modern health issues. You can purchase it in bulk, refrigerated or vacuum packed. Grind the seed in a coffee grinder and store one to two weeks' worth in the freezer. I do not recommend eating flax seed whole; it is tough on your digestive tract if not ground. This biblical seed is delicious on French toast, in oatmeal, bread, pancakes and waffles and on cereal and salads. It has a nutty flavor. If I do not put it in the morning pancakes, my nine-year-old notices and reminds me to add it. It is very inexpensive and can be stored frozen in the seed form for up to six months. Most Americans have a shortage of omega-3 oils. Eating ground flax seed or taking a daily dose of flax oil is one of the best ways to increase your omega-3 oils.

Population studies have demonstrated that people who consume a diet rich in omega-3 oils have a significantly reduced risk of developing heart disease. Results from autopsy studies have shown that the highest degree of coronary artery disease is found in individuals with the lowest concentration of omega-3 oils in their fat tissues. Individuals with the lowest degree of coronary artery disease had the highest concentrations of omega-3 oils.[10]

Hormone-free red meats are produced from cows that are not fed antibiotics, growth hormones or steroids. They cannot get mad cow disease because they are not fed the ground-up body parts of other cattle, sheep and chickens. Yes, mad cow disease has developed because stockyards are feeding the animal by-products (animal body parts that are left over after killing the animal) of dead cows, chickens and sheep to their cattle.[11] Cattle are herbivores (animals meant to eat plants). We cannot mess with God's design and feed cow by-products to cows without reaping the consequences. Free-range cattle are allowed to roam around freely and eat natural grass. Stockyard cattle are kept in tight, often crowded pens. Free-range cattle are healthier because they are getting exercise and are not locked up in close quarters so they do not spread illnesses as rapidly. If you can get grass-fed/grain-finished meat, it usually tastes the best, because as God tells us in Isaiah 32:20: *"How blessed you will be… letting your cattle…range free."* Finishing with grain before going to market enhances the flavor of the meat.

Hormone-free chickens are also not fed antibiotics, growth hormones, or steroids. Farmers will tell you that, without growth hormones, it takes twelve weeks to raise a chicken from egg to full grown and ready for market. Modern use of growth hormones has reduced that time to five and a half or six weeks! That is a reduction of almost 50 percent! Hormone-free chicken will cost you more, but it is worth it!

In its February 2006 issue, *Consumer Reports*, a magazine written by an independent testing and information organization serving only consumers, advised consumers to purchase these items in their organic (or natural) form as often as possible: meat, poultry and eggs. The reasoning is that you "greatly reduce your exposure to the agent believed to cause mad cow disease and minimize exposure to other potential toxins in non-organic feed. You also avoid the results of production methods that use daily supplemental hormones and antibiotics, which have been linked to antibacterial resistance in humans."[12]

Natural chips do not contain partially hydrogenated oil, color dyes or high fructose corn syrup. Ideally, they are not cooked at extremely high temperatures and will therefore not cause free radical damage. It is hard to identify chips cooked at lower temperatures.

While it is true there is no official United States government-regulated definition for the term "natural" pertaining to the natural food products, the FDA refers to natural ingredients as "ingredients extracted directly from plants or animal products as opposed to being produced synthetically." The USDA has a legal definition for "natural," but it applies only to meat and poultry. Those products carrying the "natural" claim must not contain any artificial flavoring. "Processed" is defined by the USDA as a process that fundamentally alters the raw product. Consumers Union, publisher of *Consumer Reports*, states, "Natural is a general claim that the product or packaging is made from or innate to the environment and that nothing artificial or synthetic has been added." There is currently no standard for the term except for meat and poultry products.[13]

I have been checking labels on products marked "natural," and have found that all the products that carry the natural label *do* adhere to the meat and poultry definition. I have not found a food labeled "natural" to have artificial ingredients.

Organic crackers and cookies do not have the forbidden partially hydrogenated oils (explained shortly), color dyes and high fructose corn syrup. Organic crackers and cookies still have sugars, but these sugars are organic and thus produced without pesticides. Some use organic cane juice, a less refined sugar. It is difficult to find cookies that fit our modernized taste buds, as we Americans like the flavor of high fructose corn syrup. It may take several attempts to find the ones your family likes. Our family has found Newman-O's to be palatable in place of name brand crème-filled cookies.

Breyer's All Natural Ice Cream in the basic flavors contains only natural ingredients and is a good substitute for other ice creams. Ice cream was one of the last things we gave up, because it is one of our favorite treats. We have decided that some foods are easier to take out of our diet; however, some foods are very important to us, and we don't want to change them. Ice cream is one of those treats that we go out for when we celebrate or "cheat."

In Phase I, there are many things to take out of your diet. These items can be very difficult to give up because we have become addicted to them and have no idea what else to eat. These foods definitely taste great. That is the goal of the manufacturer, to leave you wanting more and to have you looking for them when you are hungry. Most of them are carbohydrates and help us pack on the pounds.

It took our family about five days of withdrawal symptoms when we gave up these foods. We had eliminated many of the forbidden items but went hard-core one day and soon felt the cravings very strongly. We were tired, crabby and craving our usual foods. It was nice to be suffering all together, because it helped keep our resolve to get through those cravings. (Of course, the kids did not want me to help them get through it; they would have been happy to stop right then!)

In Phase I, you will stop purchasing or eliminate the following from your diet:

Partially hydrogenated oils wreak havoc on your body. Partial hydrogenation is a process by which food manufacturers make a liquid oil become solid at room temperature. The process of partially hydrogenating oil is what allows us to have boxed crackers, cookies and chips that stay solid even though they contain oil. It helps the crackers, cookies and chips remain on the shelf for years without breaking down. They do not taste bad either. The hydrogenation process results in cells known as free radicals. As we discussed earlier, free radicals are cells that are unstable because they are missing an electron. They bind to the electrons of healthy cells in your body and begin the process of oxygenating, or breaking down, and altering the healthy cells. This causes aging, arthritis, cancer and most of our modern illness. Omega-3 oils contain cells that fill in these loose electrons and keep our bodies healthier at a cellular level.

If these products last for years in your pantry before they mold, break down or go bad, how does your body break them down? Real food was made to mold, ferment and break down into the enzymes, minerals and vitamins your body needs to function at its best and to fight off disease.

High fructose corn syrup is yummy! It is in all my past favorite foods and probably in most of yours. Using high fructose corn syrup in foods is an inexpensive way to make foods taste sweeter than even sugar can do. That is why we like it so much. As we discussed earlier, it is terrible for your body and is one of the top items on the "forbidden list."

Vegetable oils need to be eliminated from our diets because they are usually heat-processed. This changes the molecular structure of the oils, once again, causing free radical damage.

Soft margarine has a molecular structure much like the molecular structure of the plastic container it comes in. If you put the container in your pantry or garage, bugs will not collect on it, critters will not eat it; it will not break down, and it will not grow mold. I have been storing an open container of soft tub margarine in our cabinet for two years, and the margarine has not broken down or changed at all, except to dry out. Once again, if it does not break down on the shelf, how can it break down in our bodies? Our bodies work very hard to eliminate products like this one.

White bread contains bleached flour. Bleach is not a food and is actually a poison. It never belongs in our bodies, which is why we are instructed to contact the poison control center if our child drinks it. There is nothing naturally nutritious in bleached flour, nor the white bread made from it. Any time a manufacturer has to add nutrients to a product it is selling (like "enriched" breads), we are eating fewer nutrients than we were meant to eat. When a manufacturer enriches a food, it means the manufacturer has stripped the food of most of its original nutrients and the manufacturer has tried to add back some of what it took out. Natural foods come packed with vitamins and minerals that have not been stripped out and added back. White flour and white sugar lower our immune systems and make us more susceptible to illnesses and diseases. When you get sick, look at what you ate a few days earlier. You can almost always trace your illness back to high white flour and/or white sugar intake a few days before the illness showed up. Your body's white blood cells were busy fighting off the foreign substance called bleach and did not have the white blood cells available to fight off the illness you got.

Fruits and vegetables grown with pesticides contain the poisons that keep bugs from eating them. It is not unusual for fruit and vegetable crops to be sprayed ten to fifteen times between the time they are planted and eaten.[14] These poisons are sprayed on the plants in doses low enough to kill just the little unwanted bugs, but when we eat these pesticides on our fruits and vegetables over and over again, we are getting large doses of pesticides over the course of a lifetime. When you eat thin-skinned fruits and vegetables, like apples, peaches, strawberries and cherries, you are actually eating the skin that contains most of the pesticides. In his book, *Eight Weeks to Optimum Health*, Andrew Weil cites a nonprofit organization called the Environmental Working Group that reports periodically on health risks from pesticides in produce. The group says you can cut your exposure to pesticides by 50 percent simply by reducing your consumption of the "dirty dozen"—the twelve fruits they have found to be the most contaminated. At the time of his most recent publication, those were: strawberries, bell peppers (both green and red), spinach, cherries, peaches, Mexican cantaloupes, celery, apples, apricots, green beans, Chilean grapes and cucumbers.[15] *Consumer Reports* adds pears, potatoes and red raspberries to its own dirty dozen list.[16] When purchasing any of these fruits and vegetables, make sure you buy organic. Basically, if you eat the skin of the fruit or vegetable, you ought to buy an organic one. The fruits and vegetables you eat most often are the most important ones to purchase without pesticides.

The London Food Commission conducted an in-depth study on the ingredients currently permitted for use in the manufacturing of pesticides. The results revealed that almost 40 percent of pesticides currently in use could damage the body in at least one way. Of the 426 chemicals listed, sixty-eight were found to be carcinogenic, sixty-one capable of mutating genes, thirty-five to have various reproductive effects ranging from impotence to birth defects, and ninety-three to cause skin irritations and other symptoms. Of all the studies researched by the author, the condition most frequently referred to in relation to agricultural chemicals is cancer.[17] Very often, when people have a reaction to food and think they are allergic to it, they may actually be sensitive to the pesticide used on that food.

Dryer sheets contain formaldehyde, a known carcinogen. My family lives in Colorado—one of the driest states in the nation, so eliminating dryer sheets left me concerned that we would have static cling in our clothes. I purchased a drying rack and now put all our synthetic soccer shorts and pajama-type clothes on this rack. We have not had much of a static cling problem. During the drier winter months, I have used a natural liquid fabric softener listed in the product favorites section.

CHAPTER 3

Phase II
Addressing Your Skin

In Phase II, we will address one of the most important ways to remain healthy and the first large purchase item of the process, a household water filter system. I will also begin to challenge you to think about the things going into your body that are not foods. Your skin is the largest organ of elimination. It can filter out poisons or allow poisons to enter your body, depending on what you put on it. In this phase, we will begin to replace items you use on your skin.

In Phase II, begin purchasing the following products:

        Household water filter
        Organic peanut butter
        Power bars
        Fresh ground spelt flour
        Organic deodorant and tampons
        Organic milk and cheese
        Wild cold-water fish
        Local raw honey
        Organic cold cereals and granolas
        Long-cooking oatmeal
        Organic shampoos, soaps, lotions

Organic coffee
Peppermint oil

Eliminate or avoid:

Plastic water bottles
Peanut butter with partially hydrogenated oils
Pop/soda
White flour
Farm-raised seafood without fins and scales
Non-organic boxed cereals/oatmeal/granola bars
Grocery store deodorant and tampons
Non-organic milks and cheeses
NSAID (non-steroidal anti-inflammatory drugs)
        pain relievers
Non-organic shampoos
Non-organic coffee and coffee creamers
Food containing color dyes
Lotions or soaps that contain: sodium lauryl sulfate,
        propylene glycol, color dyes

Household water filters are critical in the process of improving your health. Filters used for the entire house are costly, at an average of $1,300, but can save your pipes from needing to be replaced. (This is how my husband bought in to the whole idea.) If you are on city water, you are drinking and washing yourself in chlorine. Chlorine is highly poisonous. If you drink it straight, you are instructed to call poison control. The daily use of this poison on the inside and outside of our bodies is doing substantial damage.

The best type of water filter for under your kitchen sink is a reverse osmosis (RO) filter. A reverse osmosis water filter costs $300–$400. It stops nearly every contaminant from coming into your faucet. Most units force water first through a flashlight-size "pre-filter" that strains out sediment and then through a cellophane-like membrane that screens out even smaller pollutants. Before reaching a special faucet mounted on your sink, the now-clean water gets one last scrubbing from a carbon filter that removes any lingering chemicals picked up along the way. The main disadvantage to an RO filter is that it wastes two to four gallons of tap water for every gallon that it filters. Therefore, it is installed under your kitchen faucet. People using city water should strongly consider getting a water neutralizer and an RO filter.

While we are on the subject of water, it should be noted that virtually all the patients Dr. Gail Warner sees are dehydrated to some level. One hundred percent of the kids with attention deficit disorder/attention deficit hyperactivity disorder (ADD/ADHD) whom she sees are dehydrated. We need to be sure to drink enough purified water to help our bodies function properly. To determine the amount of water your body requires each day, divide your weight by two and drink that amount of water in ounces every day. So if you weigh 120 pounds, your body needs sixty ounces of purified water (not cola and coffee) each day. That is approximately two large polystyrene containers or eight eight-ounce glasses. We need to be sure we urinate a light yellow color.

Glass water bottles do not break down in the heat of your car. The plastic water bottles deteriorate a bit when heated or scratched and some of the plastic is released into your water. That is why your water tastes funny after it has been in your car on a hot, sunny day. Doesn't it make you wonder what prevents the containers from being heated in the transportation truck on the way to the store? Right now, even the hard plastic bottles are causing concern in the health industry. While they sort it out, I recommend using glass bottles. I often try to reuse glass containers I already have. It's better for us and hey, reusing is good for the environment, too!

Peanuts often contain mold and are full of pesticides. The national brands of peanut butter usually contain partially hydrogenated oils and thus cause free radical damage. My family's favorite brand of organic peanut butter is Maranatha, which is available at health food stores and most national chain grocery stores. It must be refrigerated after opening but tastes creamy and does not need to be remixed every time you reuse it. This peanut butter can be purchased in bulk. You can also grind you own peanut butter in a Vita Mix. How cool is that?!

Sometimes I wonder if the increase in peanut allergies today is because of allergies to the peanuts or because of allergies to the pesticides used in the growing of the peanuts.

Clif and Luna bars are our family's replacement for candy bars and most granola bars. They are the only ones I have found that taste good (even to a picky seven-year-old) and do not contain any forbidden ingredients like high fructose corn syrup, partially hydrogenated oils, etc. The Clif brand does not contain iron and is, therefore, best for boys and young girls. The Luna brand is best for teenage girls and women, as it will help replace the iron lost every month. My boys' favorite Clif bars are the brownie and chocolate chip flavors. My girls and I prefer the s'mores Luna bars.

Spelt flour is a grain like whole wheat. In the United States, it is a less popular form of wheat and, therefore, may not have been genetically altered as much as regular wheat. It contains less gluten than regular wheat and can be tolerated by some people with wheat allergies. It has more protein, good fat and fiber than wheat, and the body can more easily digest it.[18] You can use it just like wheat in recipes for pancakes, waffles and muffins and in recipes like the ones in the back of this book. You can purchase spelt flour at health food stores in bulk or prepackaged. We use it for virtually all our recipes.

Antiperspirants used by most Americans contain aluminum and propylene glycol. Aluminum has been well documented as a cause of Alzheimer's. Propylene glycol is antifreeze. It clogs the skin pores under your arms, which may be a contributing cause of breast cancer. Our underarms are a primary area for perspiration. They are designed by God to help us cool our bodies. Clogging these pores and preventing the flow of perspiration alters our body's ability to clean out poisons. When I first changed to an organic deodorant, I found that I would smell during very hot weather, for the first year, while my pores were cleaning themselves out. I have been using an organic deodorant for seven years and never have an odor problem, no matter how hot it is.

Typical tampons contain bleach. Why would a woman knowingly put bleach into the most sensitive part of her body? It causes us to cramp and bleed more. Using natural tampons reduces cramps and menstrual flow by significant amounts. This switch to natural tampons seems like it would be a costly one, but after a few months you will be paying the same price per month because even though natural tampons cost more per box, you will use fewer per month. Every month you use natural tampons, you may be pleasantly surprised by your reduced menstrual flow and fewer cramps. As you eat more of the foods God made, you may be pleasantly surprised by your reduced PMS symptoms.

Organic milk and cheese come from cows that have not been fed growth hormones or antibiotics. Antibiotic means "against life." Antibiotics kill off the good flora you need in your stomach. This lack of good flora sets the stage for many digestive problems. Growth hormones are fed to cattle to increase their size and decrease the time it takes to get a cow to market. Could there be a relationship between the amount of hormones in our food supply and the increased number of boys and girls going through early puberty?

Wild cold-water fish with fins and scales, like salmon, halibut, tuna and mackerel, contain omega-3 oils in the highest levels. They swim in the deep, cold waters of the ocean. Bottom feeders (lobster, crab and shrimp) contain high levels of mercury because they eat the trash off the bottom of the ocean. We try to eat wild, cold-water fish two to three times per week. When I order fish in a restaurant, I ask the waiter if the fish is farm raised or wild before I decide to order. Most restaurant fish is farm raised. Farm-raised fish do not swim in the ocean and, therefore, are not getting the exercise they need to stay healthy. In addition, the color of farm-raised salmon is often enhanced with color dyes.

Local raw honey can help reduce allergies just like the "hair of the dog that bit you." The theory is that honey grown local to the area you live has small doses of the airborne allergies you may have. This should help reduce your sensitivities to those allergies just like the small doses of shots the allergist gives to help build up immunities to the allergen. If the honey is raw, it has not been heated, and thus the enzymes and minerals have not been destroyed. Honey is still sugar and thus raises your blood sugar levels, but it is not refined and is the type of sugar that God meant it to be. After all, God brought the Israelites to the "land of milk and honey."

Organic cold cereals and granola do not contain pesticides or high fructose corn syrup. This is important because wheat is full of pesticides. Cereal crops receive an average of eight applications of chemicals between the time they are planted and eaten.[19] If you can find organic cereal that you and your children like, rest assured they will not be eating pesticides, nor will they be getting color dyes or high fructose corn syrup. It can take a while for kids to adjust their taste buds to organic cereals. They have spent many years enjoying the cereals with high fructose corn syrup. Give them time; if they do not like the new cereal taste at first, wait and try again after they have eaten healthy for a while. Their taste buds will adjust. My kids' favorite choices are listed in the Product Favorites section of this book.

Long-cooking oatmeal is also known as oat groats and can be purchased in bulk. When you buy this kind of oatmeal, it will look much like whole wheat grain. Just grind it in your blender and cook it on the stovetop with two parts water to one part oat groats, for about twenty minutes. (See recipes in the back.) It is delicious and tastes great with butter and honey. Eating your oatmeal this way takes a little longer to prepare, but provides you with the micronutrients from the whole grain. The faster oatmeal is to prepare at home, the more processed it is. More processing, of course, means less nutrition than God meant for us.

Organic shampoos, soaps and lotions are critical to improving your health because, remember, skin is the biggest organ of elimination and absorption. Thus, it can absorb or eliminate vast amounts of toxins into or out of your body. We enter the shower every day and turn on the warm water, which opens the pores of our skin. We then apply shampoos and soaps that contain cancer-causing agents like sodium lauryl sulfate, EDTA and my personal favorite, propylene glycol, otherwise known as antifreeze. These products are absorbed into your skin and then into your bloodstream. They are poisons, but we all like the way products foam and lather, so we unknowingly buy them and add to the onslaught of poisons in our bodies every day.

My family's favorite shampoo and soap recommendations can be found in the reference section on Product Favorites. When our family gave up the poisonous soaps, our skin began to feel softer than it ever had before. The organic soaps cost substantially more than the soaps we are used to, but they last three to four times longer and if left on your skin they do not make you itch.

Organic coffee is made without pesticides. If you drink coffee every day, you may want to consider purchasing an organic brand. It tastes wonderful.

Peppermint oil can be used to relieve a headache. On the rare occasion that someone in our house gets a headache, we do not use typical over-the-counter pain relievers. We use peppermint oil to alleviate the pain. The oil is rubbed on the individual's temples, being careful not to get it too close to the eyes. [20] The headache often returns after ten minutes, but we rub the oil on the temples again and the headache does not return. We then increase the individual's water intake, as headaches are often a sign of mild dehydration.

We also use peppermint oil to clear a stuffy nose and help ease the sleep of someone with a cold. To apply, I rub olive oil on the individual's chest, then rub the peppermint oil on top of the olive oil. It feels great. The olive oil reduces the tingling effect.

Pop/soda is not only full of sugar, which impairs your immune system, it is also full of color dyes. Color dyes have been known to cause ADD and impotence. The carbonation pulls the calcium out of your bones. Pop has been nicknamed "osteoporosis in a can." Carbonation causes calcium loss in the bones through a three-stage process:
   1. The carbonation irritates the stomach.
   2. The stomach tries to cure the irritation by secreting the only antacid at its disposal—calcium. It gets this calcium from the blood.
   3. The blood, now low on calcium, replenishes its supply from the bones. If it did not do this, muscular and brain function

would be severely impaired.[21]
Osteoporosis has been shown to be five times worse in kids and women who drink cola than in those who drink other types of soda. Growing children and women at risk for osteoporosis should never have pop. Our family has come to prefer water with lemon and we ask for it at restaurants. You may even go a step further and order bottled water.

White flour has the same effect on your blood sugar levels that white sugar has. They both cause blood sugar levels in our blood stream to rise quickly, producing a heightened release of insulin. Sugar and white flour both have a detrimental effect on mood, premenstrual syndrome and many other health conditions.[22] White flour is bleached; therefore, your body has to fight off the toxins and is then not equipped to fight infections that come your way, resulting in a suppressed immune system. We eliminated pretzels and many other white flour products from our diet without much hassle. The hardest part is still going to a restaurant and not eating the warm loaf of bread offered before the meal.

NSAID (non-steroidal anti-inflammatory drugs) are pain relievers. You know, the pills we take for aches, pains and headaches. They kill off the good flora in your stomach. Some of the children's versions of NSAIDs contain aspartame. Aspartame is a low-calorie flavor enhancer. It is often marketed as NutraSweet, Equal and Spoonful. It is in children's pain relievers. In her book, *Sweet Poison*, Dr. Janet Starr Hull states that the side effects from aspartame can occur gradually, can be immediate or can be acute reactions. The list of adverse reactions and side effects from aspartame is long. A small sample includes epileptic seizures, headaches, migraines, dizziness, depression, anxiety, chest palpitations, multiple sclerosis, ADD, lupus, etc. This list goes on and on.[23] Dr. Starr Hull's book also recommends how to detoxify your body from aspartame. Peppermint oil is a great substitute for headache pills. Ginger, turmeric, willow bark and peppermint oil can be used to prevent inflammation. I just rub peppermint oil on my aches and pains. It tingles, smells good and takes away the pain. Health food stores have reference books to help with correct doses and applications.

Do you see the pattern? If it tastes great, something has probably been added to enhance the flavor. We need to adjust our taste buds to enjoy the foods our bodies need. It sounds impossible to change our taste buds and actually enjoy the healthy foods. But I am here to tell you: *it is possible!* We actually enjoy and sometimes crave the foods that God made. If we can do it, you can too!

Eliminating foods that contain **color dyes** will eliminate candy from your diet—surely going to be a tough sell for your kids. Michelle, a friend from church suggested having our children bring home the goodies they receive at soccer games, school parties and the like. They place the candy in a jar in the pantry. When the jar is full, I give them five dollars, empty the jar and start over. This has helped give my younger children a reason not to eat the junk food.

Our second child had gotten into trouble several times at school and in his sports practices in elementary school. In middle school, we took him off the sugary products containing color dyes. The teachers in middle school absolutely loved him. When I told the middle school teachers and principal that he had been a "problem" child in elementary school, they couldn't believe it. Likewise, when I told the elementary teachers that he was now respected and admired by his middle school teachers, they could not believe it either. The only things we changed were his diet and prayer. Allergic reactions to color dyes have been implicated in the rise of ADHD in children. The theory that food additives, like color dyes, induce hyperactivity is commonly referred to as the "Feingold hypothesis," stemming from the research of

Benjamin Feingold, M.D.
According to Feingold, many hyperactive children—perhaps 40–50 percent—are sensitive to artificial food colors, flavors and preservatives (as we all should probably be). They are also sensitive to naturally occurring salicylates and phenolic compounds. Feingold based his claims on his experience with over 1,200 cases in which food additives were linked to learning and behavioral disorders. Other countries have significantly restricted the use of artificial food additives because of the possible harmful side effects. Several more studies have shown a relationship between the common yellow dye tartrazine and the behavior of hyperactive children.[24] We can't forget Dr Gail Warner's personal research indicating that virtually all children she treats with ADD/ADHD are dehydrated. I believe my son was one of those kids whose body could not deal with the color dyes. Now that he is off them (and taking flax oil), he is an entirely different boy!

One day I commented to this same child, "You and your brother and sisters are much easier now that we've eaten healthy for a while." He looked up and replied, "And so are you, Mom!" Taking white flour, white sugar, color dyes and other poisons out of our diet has noticeably improved the overall mood at our house.

CHAPTER 4

Phase III
Bread Machines and Lunch Meats

In Phase III, we are getting into more time-consuming ways to improve your health. I will suggest the best (and usually the most time-consuming) method to improve your health. Where possible, I will provide a faster (and perhaps slightly less ideal) method to achieve almost the same results. If you cannot do the more involved methods described here, have no guilt! Just do as my father used to say: "Do what you can and can the rest." If you are changing over to half the suggestions in this book, you are much healthier than you were before you read it, right? Feel good about that and add the more difficult processes later, if you want to and if they fit into your lifestyle.

In Phase III you will purchase or increase the following:

> Goat's milk and cheese
> Bread machine
> Pro-biotics
> Maple syrup or agave nectar
> Organic lemons
> Hormone/Nitrate-free lunch meat
> Organic condiments
> Exposure to fresh, clean air
> Deep breathing
> Exercise
> Good attitude

Eliminate or avoid the following:

> Cow's milk
> Pancake syrup
> Lunch meats/salami/pepperoni
> Bacon/pork products
> All fast food
> Artificial sweeteners

Goat's milk does not taste as bad as it sounds. It has a slightly sweeter flavor than cow's milk. I recommend starting by using it in place of cow's milk in all your recipes. No one at my house has ever noticed. (I usually tell them what I've put into the recipe after I find out if they like it.) Goat's milk is actually easy on your digestive system. Cow's milk is very difficult to digest and completely intolerable for many people. After all, there is really one purpose for cow's milk—to take a 30-pound calf and grow it into a 300-pound cow in a six-month period. With young children, you can use goat's milk on their cereal by starting with a mix of one-quarter goat's milk to three-quarters cow's milk and gradually increasing the ratio of goat's milk until you reach 100 percent goat's milk. Goat's cheese is delicious and very easy on your digestive tract. It's expensive, but we love it for a special treat. Almond and cashew milk are delicious and are explained later.

You may notice that I have not recommended using soy milk. I have read many articles containing information on soy products. The data seems inconclusive. I have not found the word "soy" in the Bible, and thus am not willing to bet my health on it. Ninety nine percent of the soy we consume is genetically modified. Soy causes mucus in our digestive tract and is a phytoestrogen, causing our bodies to make more estrogen.

In Phase III, it is time to look into purchasing a **bread machine.** Making bread is not as hard as it sounds. I start with the whole grain of wheat (my favorite is spelt flour) in the whole grain form as it is picked off the plant, grind it up and make bread. With the Bosch bread machine, I can make four loaves of bread in one hour. That is start to finish, hot bread on the counter and the kitchen all cleaned up. Spelt flour is an excellent source of phytonutrients like vitamins B1, B2, B3, copper and manganese. [25] It has a slightly sweeter, nuttier flavor than regular wheat flour, but is somewhat more crumbly. If your family is not happy going to spelt, you may want to start with a blend of hard white wheat and slowly transition to the spelt bread. Research reported at the American Institute for Cancer Research (AICR) International Conference on Food, Nutrition and Cancer, by Rui Hai Liu, M.D., Ph.D., and his colleagues at Cornell University shows that whole grains, such as spelt, contain many phytonutrients that may lower the risk for colon cancer. There seems to be a relationship between the fiber and the phytonutrients in whole grains. [26] That is why I try to use whole grain spelt flour in all my pancakes, muffins, breads, etc.

Another great product is a Vita Mix. This wonderful product has several uses, as you will see throughout this book. It may be used to grind the above mentioned grain, or used to juice delicious fruits and make healthy shakes. It retails for around $500 and is very versatile.

Making bread for your family is one of the most time-consuming tasks in the quest to eat healthier. If you choose not to make the bread, you may still purchase Rudy's bread and switch over to the Rudy spelt bread. It is not as tasty as homemade and has been sitting on the shelf longer, but it is a good substitute. Another good substitute is the Ezekiel bread. It has some advantages that even the fresh spelt does not have. Another source of whole grain bread is the Great Harvest or similar stores.

The Bosch bread maker, grain mill and miscellaneous supplies will cost approximately $400. If your family eats two loaves of good bread a week at $3.50 a loaf, you are spending $364 per year on bread. Your bread maker will pay for itself in just over one year. I believe it is important to eat grains and their bread shortly after you grind them because the nutrients are quickly lost after the grain has been ground. When archeologists opened an ancient tomb and found whole grains, they tested the grain for nutrients and found the whole grain contained all the nutrients that our wheat does today. Seventy-two hours after they cracked the grain open, it contained almost no nutrients. When God packages something, it lasts much longer than the same food does after we "open" it. So for my family of six, it is worth my time to make bread once or twice a week so they can get the micro nutrients packed in the whole grains. As you can see from the bread recipe in the back, I also add ground flax to the bread to make sure my family gets their daily dose of flax.

If you have a smaller family and don't need to make a large quantity of bread, you can use a one-loaf bread maker. There are many grain grinders on the market to choose from. If you have a Champion Juicer, you can get an attachment to grind grain for around $70.

You may choose to order only the grain mill for approximately $220. With this appliance, you can grind spelt or other grains for waffles, pancakes, muffins, cookies, etc. I substitute the fresh ground spelt flour straight across the board for regular flour and have not had any problems, except in cookies. In cookies, it helps to use half whole grain flour and half organic white flour. Many recipes are included in the recipe section. At my daughter's slumber party I made the healthy waffles for her friends and have heard they continue to ask their parents to make them just like mine.

Maple syrup is a great substitute for regular table syrup. It is more expensive and sometimes difficult for children to get used to the taste. If you find this to be a problem, you may use the recipe in the back for table syrup. The recipe is made with refined white sugar, but at least it does not contain our enemy—high fructose corn syrup. Girls at the aforementioned slumber party, and even visiting teenagers loved it. Pure cane juice can be substituted for white sugar to improve the healthiness of the syrup. If you are purchasing maple syrup, choose grades B or C as they have been refined less than grade A maple syrup.

Pro-biotics mean "for life". They are the little good germs that your stomach and digestive tract need to win the war against all the bad germs. The SAD (Standard American Diet) of processed foods causes your body to grow what we like to call bad flora. We need to put in lots of good flora to make sure we maintain a healthy balance in our gut.

Agave nectar is another substitute for table syrup. It is more fluid than honey and has a slightly more syrupy taste. It is still a sugar, but because it comes in a more natural state than white sugar or high fructose corn syrup.

The juice from organic lemons can be put into your water to improve the flavor of your water, help digestion and reduce the acid levels in your stomach. We order water with lemon, no ice, at restaurants instead of pop. Room temperature water is easier for your body to process than cold water. While we are on the subject of water again, I'd like to tell you that it is better for you to drink water between meals rather than with meals. Water dilutes the stomach acids your body produces (and needs) to help you digest your food. We try to drink most of our water about twenty minutes before or after meals. Doing things this way is not as overwhelming as it sounds; just do a little changing at a time and reread sections of this book when you are ready for more information.

Hormone- and nitrate-free lunch meats are available at deli counters at your local health food stores and in the packaged section of some grocers. Nitrates and nitrites have been associated with stomach cancer. They are abundant in lunch meats. When I cannot find nitrate/nitrite- and hormone-free lunch meats at regular supermarket delis, I request them. If enough of us request healthier foods, retailers will eventually listen.

Organic condiments are free of high fructose corn syrup and partially hydrogenated oils. If you use a condiment often, be sure to find a healthy substitute. Check the labels. You will be surprised which condiments have the "forbidden" foods. Ketchup and mayonnaise have high fructose corn syrup. Ranch dressing has monosodium glutamate.

Good clean air is essential to your health. If you do not live in the city, shut off your air conditioner, and open your windows and doors and enjoy the air the way God meant it to be. My children often get yelled at to "leave the door open; we need the fresh air." In the winter, turn off the heat on the warmer days and open the doors for a little while. It will keep you healthier.

Take time to **breathe deeply** every day. When I feel an illness coming on, I try to remember to breathe deeply several times during the day. Many times the illness never takes hold. Breathing deeply provides all your cells with oxygen needed to operate more efficiently.

Moderate exercise is critical to staying healthy. Jesus told us to be like Him. In His time, people walked everywhere they went. They did not have cars. As Kevin Trudeau reminds us in his book, *Natural Cures They Don't Want You to Know,* it helps your mental attitude if you look up while you walk. Look off at the horizon; it can't hurt![27]

We cannot forget how important our **mental attitude** is to our health. We can change our blood pressure, stomach acid and adrenalin levels just by what we think. Try it. You can get yourself all worked up just sitting here, right now. By contrast, you can also reduce your blood pressure and improve the way your immune system functions by thinking positively and staying relaxed. Use your mind to help keep yourself healthy. Remember that in Philippians 4:4-9 Jesus reminds us, *"Do not be anxious about anything, but in everything, by prayer and petition, with thanksgiving, present your requests to God. And the peace of God, which transcends all understanding, will guard your hearts and your mind in Christ Jesus. Finally, brothers, whatever is true, whatever is noble, whatever is right, whatever is pure, whatever is lovely, whatever is admirable—if anything is excellent or praiseworthy—think about such things. Whatever you have learned or received or heard from me, or seen in me—put it into practice. And the peace of God will be with you."*

Bacon and pork products are on God's "do not eat" list in Leviticus 11:1-8. Scientists continue to agree with God's instructions that the pork products we eat today are not good for us. They contain nitrates and nitrites used to preserve, prevent the growth of microorganisms and add color. They have been implicated in a variety of long-term health problems, including cancer.[28]

It is now time to eliminate **fast food** from your diet. This one is tough for us Americans. We live in a fast-paced world and like our food to be the same. Due to pressure from the consumer, this industry is starting to change, but most fast-food restaurants still use the highly processed, high-temperature oils we are trying to eliminate from your diet. They often use high fructose corn syrup. There is nothing naturally nutritious in the white flour buns. The French fries do not have enough potatoes in them to count as a vegetable. Have you ever lost a fast-food French fry in the crevice of your car and found it months later only to discover that it looks just like it did the day you bought it? At our house, we have been storing an open container of French fries in our pantry for two years. Other than being a little drier, they look just like they did the day I put them there. How do our bodies break these foods down? Food should grow mold and go bad when it is not eaten. It is this deteriorating quality about food that allows our bodies to digest food and break it down into useable forms.

When my oldest son was a toddler, I was so proud to have him eat his first Happy Meal that I actually took a picture of him while he ate it. We used to go to fast-food restaurants at least once a week. When this same son was not growing or gaining weight, I took him to doctors who told me he was allergic to wheat, corn and dairy. Because we were on the SAD (Standard American Diet) at the time, roughly all his food contained wheat, corn or dairy. Because he was allergic to so much of his diet, his body was spending virtually all its energy trying to digest food. He was losing weight and looked like a child with "failure to thrive" syndrome. We took him off fast food, changed all our diets to Phase I, and took him to a chiropractor who eliminated his allergies. In a few years, he has gained sixty-five pounds and nine inches. He has improved his skin color, energy level and athletic performance dramatically.

Our family has been off fast food for roughly seven years. At first it was difficult to take the time to go to a sit-down restaurant while we were traveling. But we found that it did not add much time to the trip, and we enjoyed the down time together. We also discovered that we did not have the mood swings and reduction in energy level roughly two hours after the meal as we had noticed after eating fast-food meals.

Artificial sweeteners are Equal, NutraSweet, Spoonful and Splenda, etc. The list of adverse effects linked to these sweeteners is enormous, as stated earlier. It includes non-Hodgkin's lymphoma, hypothyroidism, Graves' disease, chronic fatigue syndrome, frequency of voiding and burning during urination, marked thinning of hair, hives, and abdominal pain.[29] Read Dr. Janet Hull's book, *Sweet Poison* for more information and for instructions on how to detoxify from these poisons.

CHAPTER 5

Phase IV
Nuts, Condiments and Bug Spray

In Phase IV, you will begin or purchase the following:

> Almond milk
> Raw nuts
> More raw fruits and vegetables
> Experimentation with separating your foods
> Pure Cane Juice/Stevia
> Herbal teas
> Organic onions and garlic
> Aluminum-free baking powder and tortillas
> Sea salt/Celtic salt
> Organic seasoning mixes
> Organic bug spray

You will eliminate or reduce the following:

> Table salt/baking powder/tortillas with aluminum
> Cooked and vacuum-sealed nuts
> Non-organic packaged seasoning mixes and
> condiments
> Bug spray with DEET
> Potatoes and corn
> Aluminum foil
> Chewing gum

Almond milk tastes even better than goat's milk and can be interchanged with goat's milk or regular milk in any recipe. It contains calcium and other nutrients and will not cause the phlegm buildup that cow's milk causes. It is often sweetened, so do not overuse it. The chocolate version makes a great hot chocolate. Even the teenagers who don't like our health food enjoy this hot chocolate.

You can even make your own almond milk using the Vita Mix mentioned earlier.

Raw nuts are healthier for you than cooked nuts because, once again, the raw version of a food contains the enzymes our bodies need to digest that food. Many cooked nuts that come in vacuum-sealed jars contain sugars and MSG (monosodium glutamate).

MSG is a flavor enhancer. It is made from an industrial fermentation process. John Erb, a research assistant at the University of Waterloo, Ontario, Canada, discovered that scientists had created a new "race" of experimental rats called "MSG-Treated Rats." These rats are consistently obese. These morbidly obese rats are created by injecting them with MSG when they are born. The MSG triples the amount of insulin that the pancreas creates, causing rats (and humans?) to become obese.[30] People are often allergic to MSG and do not know it.

My sister uses raw walnuts in her cookies. She grinds them in a coffee grinder or food processor and just adds them to her cookies. Her children have never noticed. Walnuts are rich with omega-3 oils, which help prevent cancer and the effects of aging.

Increase your consumption of **raw fruits and vegetables**. All raw foods have those wonderful enzymes our bodies need to digest the foods we eat. Cooking these same foods reduces the enzymes they contain. Fifty percent of our diets (by sight, not by weight) should consist of fruits and vegetables. Try eating fruits and vegetables for breakfast. I enjoy sautéing onions and eating them with eggs for breakfast. Remember to emphasize the organic leafy green vegetables we learned about in school, like broccoli, celery, spinach and lettuce. When eating salads with all these great vegetables, I add flax oil to the salad dressing I am using. I can't taste it and I am getting my one tablespoon a day the easy way.

Experiment with **separating your foods** as you eat them. This means eating fruits at one sitting and then waiting thirty minutes, eating grains at another meal, waiting two hours, and eating meats at another sitting. Again, wait two hours before eating other types of foods. This allows your stomach to produce the appropriate digestive enzymes for each food category. It reduces stomach pains and eases digestion. Vegetables can be eaten with any other food. *The Raw Food Detox Diet* by nutritionist Natalie Rose explains this approach to food.[31] It is a completely different way of life but allows you to better digest your food and will help you feel much healthier.

Pure Cane Juice is the unrefined sugar off the cane plant. It is still sugar and will raise your blood sugar level, but it is less refined than white sugar and is not bleached. **Stevia** is a natural form of sugar; it can be used to replace sugar in your recipes and drinks.

Herbal teas are a great substitute for coffee. At one point in my life, I was drinking up to six cups of coffee a day. If someone that addicted to caffeine can make the switch to herbal teas, you can too. With tea, I still get that "International Moment" feeling, but I am actually getting health benefits from my drink. Ginger and peppermint teas are good for digestion, chamomile tea will help you sleep and relax, and dandelion tea is a detox aid. Detox aids help remove poisons from your body. I recommend choosing organic teas to continue to reduce your exposure to pesticides.

Organic onion and garlic will boost your immune system. They also help kill off the bad flora in your digestive track. I add them to all the dishes I can. On the rare days that I do feel a cold coming on, I put a clove of garlic in my cheek for as long as I can stand it. Sometimes the cold goes away within hours. Some of my kids (as young as seven) have been able to do this. Their colds also go away very quickly.[32] Garlic is especially effective in the healing of sinus infections and runny noses.

Aluminum causes Alzheimer's disease. It is added to most grocery store tortillas. It is also used in table salt and baking powder to keep them from clumping. **Sea salt** (our favorites are REAL Salt and Celtic Salt) does not contain aluminum and has an added bonus of extra trace minerals our bodies need. You will need to get used to the clumping and just stir it loose when you use it, since sea salt does not have aluminum to keep it from clumping.

Packaged seasoning mixes and condiments often contain MSG, high fructose corn syrup or partially hydrogenated oils. The instant and packaged products we purchase often have these poisons in their ingredients lists to increase the flavor, ensure that the product lasts many months on the shelf, and make it easier for us to prepare. If your family is attached to a particular condiment brand, it may be difficult to switch them to an organic version. My family has still not found an acceptable organic version of ranch dressing or mayonnaise. We have found the Hunt's Organic Ketchup and the Muir Glen Organic Ketchup to be very tasty. As a general rule, if you use the condiment or packaged seasoning mix often, it is worth it to find a substitute.

Bug spray contains the poison DEET. If a product is poison to one life form, it most likely is poison to all life forms in varying degrees. Instead of using DEET, you can use organic bug sprays that contain lavender and rosemary, which are naturally occurring bug repellents, but not poisons.

Potatoes and corn are foods that God created, but we humans have genetically altered them over and over again to increase crop yields and improve resistance to pests. They, like wheat, have been altered so many times they are no longer on most experts' recommended lists of foods.

Aluminum foil needs to be eliminated from our food-storage uses because the aluminum leaches into the foods it touches and has been attributed to the increase in Alzheimer's disease.

Chewing gum often contains aspartame. There are digestive gums available in health food stores that do not last as long as other gums but can aid in digestion and do not taste bad. Our favorites are listed in the Product Favorites section.

CHAPTER 6

Phase V
Cooking, Lymph Nodes, Candles and Chiropractors

In Phase V, you will begin or purchase the following:

> Pressing/dry brushing your lymph nodes
> Practicing body massage
> Looking for a doctor of chiropractic
> Making bread crumbs and croutons
> Getting juice fasting supplies
> Consuming green drinks
> Using organic sun screen/makeup/"natural" nail polish
> Buying organic candles
> Using laundry /dish soap without phosphates or dyes
> Using stainless steel pots/pans/spatulas
> Using glass jars for food storage
> Buying supplements
> Brushing with natural toothpaste

You will eliminate or reduce the following:

> Petroleum products
> Non-organic sun screen/makeup/nail polish
> Non-organic candles
> Perfume
> Your microwave

Laundry and dish soap with phosphates and dyes
Non-stick pans and spatulas
Plastic food-storage dishes
Household chemicals

In Phase V, we begin to improve the household and cooking environment by further eliminating chemicals and plastics that are damaging to our bodies. I will also challenge you to think about going out of your comfort zone and looking into alternative care for your body.

Your **lymph system** collects poisons and eliminates them. You have many lymph nodes throughout your body, including those along both sides of your spine, the outside of your legs, the inside of your arms, in your groin (yes, sex among married couples is good for us!), at the top of your neck, and under your chin. When any of your lymph nodes are overloaded, they will swell (just as when you have a swollen neck along with a sore throat). Pressing your lymph nodes helps keep them clean and flowing thus preventing illnesses. During the winter, we try to rub the lymph nodes along each family member's spine to help ward off colds and illness. It's one more thing that can't hurt and makes us feel better.

Lymph nodes can also be aided by **dry brushing**. To dry brush, you purchase a natural bristle brush at your local health food store and brush your dry skin before you shower. Brush gently from the limbs toward the heart, as the lymph system drains toward the heart. Since I started adding this to my routine, my skin feels softer than it did in high school.

Body massage is another good way to keep the lymph system clean; and hey, it feels good too!

I was raised in a traditional family that went to the doctor when we were sick and took our prescription medicine if necessary.

I thought **chiropractors** were "quacks." I have since realized that the basic system of thought behind chiropractic care is what I was taught in high school biology. Remember when we were taught in science that all nerves run from the brain, down your spine to all your limbs, organs and muscles? These nerves communicate to the voluntary and involuntary muscles so our bodies run properly. When we injure any of these nerves running down the spine, we can become paralyzed or die because critical communication cannot happen between the brain and our organs or muscles. It's like having a bad connection on a cell phone call; the information just can't get through unless the lines of communication are clear. Chiropractic care keeps small pinches and kinks that occur through daily living from preventing the proper function of our organs. Keeping the spine in alignment will prevent pinches in this communication system and allow our bodies to run as they were meant to run.

Going to a doctor of chiropractic care is a sensitive subject for many. It is an individual decision, as are all the choices suggested in this book. As you pick and choose which items in each phase work for you, I hope you give chiropractic care a consideration. Make sure you talk to people and find a reputable one. Just as in any profession, there are good chiropractors and poor chiropractors. Finding a good one can mean the difference between solving some chronic health issues and continuing to take medicine to cover up those health issues.

Juice fasts are a great way to kick-start your way to improved health. To conduct a juice fast, purchase a good quality juicer and follow the instructions to consume no solids—only diluted fresh juices for one or more days, depending on the severity of your health issues and the amount of cleansing you desire. For around $250, you can purchase a good quality juicer. See the Resources section for recommendations. Juice fasting gives your digestive system a chance to stop processing food and clean itself out. Leafy green vegetables are the healthiest foods to juice but may be difficult to enjoy. You may want to add some fruit or sweet vegetables like carrots to your juice to make them more palatable. Many people add colonics and enemas to their fasting regime to further improve their health.

Be careful to fast on days when you can get some rest and be sure to get enough fluids. I did a fast that almost landed me in the hospital because I did not pay enough attention to my fluid intake. Even with that mistake, I felt substantially better after the fast than I did before the fast. When you finish a juice fast, you need to be very careful to slowly go back to eating. When you return to a normal diet too quickly and with the wrong foods, you can cause severe stomach aches and illness. A general rule of thumb is that you should take half as many days you spent on the fast to return to full eating. For more on this subject, I recommend reading *Cleansing Made Simple* by Cheryl Townsley, N.D. [33]

As we have been taught for years, the **leafy green vegetables** are the healthiest foods available to us. Green drinks are basically condensed, dry green vegetables that you can drink. Some of the better-tasting ones are Nano Greens, Earth's Promise and Isagenix Ionix Supreme.

You can grow your own vegetables to ensure you get the least expensive, freshest vegetables available. Getting your vegetables from the garden to the table in the fastest manner possible gives you the best chance of getting the most vitamins from your veggies. Therefore, homegrown is the best. Another good source for vegetables is to purchase them from local farmers' markets and/or buy them local and in season.

Organic sunscreen does not contain EDTA, parabens or other toxins but is still very effective in guarding against the sun's damage. It needs to be applied at least twenty minutes before you go into the water and right after you get out, as it will wash off skin easily.

Non-organic makeup contains all kinds of products that we would not put on our skin if we were aware of what is in the ingredients list. It can have all the usual poisons like pesticides, propylene glycol, EDTA and even lead. Some also contain petroleum products and bone meal, which is the crushed bone of animals.

Nail polish and nail polish removers do not come in a "natural" form, but they do come with fewer poisons when purchased at health food stores. Some of the things to watch out for and try to avoid in nail polish and removers are ethyl acetate and acetone. The more natural versions tend to flake off your nails more easily than their more poisonous counterparts.

The wax in candles is a petroleum product. Petroleum products contain "xenoestrogens," which means the fumes they give off have an estrogen-like impact on our body tissues. Too much estrogen has been cited as a cause of breast cancer.[34] Natural candles made of bee's wax and natural fragrances are much more expensive than candles made of petroleum products, so I purchase both but use the toxic candles for decoration and burn only the natural candles.

Laundry and dishwasher soaps contain toxins like phosphates that are not good for septic tanks or for our bodies. When we rub against or ingest the residue on our clothes and dishes, we are adding to the onslaught of poisons for our bodies to eliminate. However, natural soaps do not remove stains as well as some brand-name products. You may want to hang on to one bottle of the old laundry soap to help get out those stubborn stains. I try to use bleach only when absolutely necessary.
Stainless steel pans do not contain the aluminum found in

nonstick pans. PFOA, an ingredient in Teflon, has been found in the blood of 95 percent of tested Americans. It has been tied to cancer and developmental damage in animal studies. It is used in the process that makes stain-, grease- and water-resistant products including microwave popcorn bags, pizza box liners, nonstick cookware, pillows, upholstery and carpet. Industrial giant DuPont agreed in December 2005 to pay $10.25 million in fines for research and education to resolve federal charges that it hid information about the dangers posed by PFOA.[35] Stainless steel pans are a great alternative. They last a long time and come in a range of prices. The Teflon in our nonstick pots, pans and utensils peels and rubs off and gets into our food; so even if you are making an organic meal, you may be adding poison to it if you are using these products.

Glass jars do not outgas like their plastic counterparts do. Plastic contains petroleum and when heated to a high temperature, the plastic can leach into your food. I wash and reuse glass jars from other foods (like the Maranatha peanut butter jars). We still use plastic, as it is very difficult to get away from it; we just try to keep its use to a minimum. If you continue to use plastic food containers, be sure not to microwave or heat foods in them, as high heat can cause the plastic to leach into your food. I also continue to use plastic bags to pack my kids' lunches because I have not found a better alternative.

Supplements may be very helpful in restoring your health or they may be a waste of money. It depends on the quality of the supplements. However, there are no regulations for supplements. This keeps the costs down, but it also means the buyer must beware. It can be difficult to know if you are getting a quality product. For the most part, it is best to use pharmaceutically tested vitamins and supplements.

One way to verify the quality of a supplement is to check the label. For a quick check, you can add the total milligrams (mgs) from all the ingredients listed on the back of the container and see if the total quantity of mgs exceeds the total quantity of mgs on the front of the container. The total milligrams from the list of ingredients cannot possibly be more than the total mgs in the whole vitamin.

Doctor Gail Warner has X-rayed many people and seen the shape of many vitamins on the X-rays. Invariably, she asks people if they are taking grocery store daily vitamins and the answer is yes. A quick check I use to see if the vitamins will break down in our bodies is to put one in water. If it dissolves, it is sure to break down in our stomachs.

Natural toothpaste that tastes good was very difficult to find. It took over a year and almost twenty different tries before I found ones my family will use. We have found Nature's Gate's Herbal Crème Natural Toothpaste, Cool Mint Gel Natural Toothpaste and Natural Whitening Gel Dental Therapy to be ones we are willing to use. They still took some getting used to, and we have to be careful when we squeeze some of the tubes not to break a hole in them, but they are worth it. Have you ever read the ingredients on a national brand of toothpaste? It says "do not ingest."

Fluoride may cause people to become passive. Because of this it was used to sedate prisoners of war who were in concentration camps. Their passive behaviors kept them from trying to escape and from caring that they were in captivity.

If you still have ambitions to do even more to keep your family healthy at this point, you can start saving your **bread crusts and heels**, storing them in the refrigerator, and using them to make Kathy Weiler's breadcrumbs and croutons listed in the recipe section. It is very rewarding to know that even the bread crumbs and croutons we eat are helping us get healthier.

Perfume smells wonderful but may be dangerous to our health. In a September 16, 1986, report by the Committee on Science & Technology, U.S. House of Representatives, it was revealed that 95 percent of chemicals used in fragrances are synthetic compounds derived from petroleum (which we remember is an xenoestrogen and causes our bodies to produce estrogen). These chemical compounds include benzene derivatives, aldehydes and many other known toxins and sensitizers capable of causing cancer, birth defects, central nervous system disorders and allergic reactions.[36]

There are 62,000 results of an Internet search regarding the dangers of **microwave** cooking. Several of them discuss a situation where a nurse heated a patient's blood transfusion in a microwave before administering it. The patient died. Have you noticed how you would not want to eat a steak from the microwave? It looks nothing like its grilled counterpart. Butter melted in the microwave looks very different from butter melted on the stove. We have had many heated discussions at our house about the scientific reasoning behind the potential dangers of microwaves. To compromise, we have installed an Advantium oven. It is the same size and shape as a microwave oven, it is placed in the same spot in the kitchen and it does three functions: convection cooking, "traditional" microwave cooking (which we try not to use), and speed cooking, which does most of the cooking with light and just finishes with microwaves (we try to shut it off before it switches to microwaves). We also just try to heat more things right on the stove top or in the toaster oven. It takes awhile to get back into the habit of heating water for tea on the stove, etc., but once you get the old habits back, it is no big deal.

Household chemicals are an obvious form of toxins in our environment, but in a person's quest to keep a clean house, we are unsure which ones we can eliminate. Start by using the natural pump soaps at your sinks. We need to use non-anti-bacterial soaps because continued use of antibacterial soaps just builds up the various bacteria's resistance to the soaps. You can also stop using chemicals to clean windows and glass. Water and paper towels work just as well, or you can purchase a *Magic Cloth* online at www.magiccloth.com for about $12. I have also found a cheaper version of the Magic Cloth at my local dollar store. You can use this cloth to clean windows, glass, counters and appliances and to dust furniture. This product alone will eliminate many harsh chemicals you are using and breathing. I also use it with warm soap and water to clean my sinks. It works like, well, magic.

My neighbor uses baking soda and water to clean her toilets. The baking soda provides the abrasive needed to get the tough dirt.

CHAPTER 7

You Can Do It!

The closer we get to eating food the way God made it, the better that food is for us. Raw food is better for us than cooked food. Fresh food is better than frozen; and we should avoid canned, processed and packaged foods. We can try to violate many of God's laws, including His laws about food and what we put in our bodies, but the consequences will always come back to get us in a negative way. Violating any of God's laws is like trying to violate God's law of gravity. You can disagree with His law of gravity, believe it applies to only some people, claim it is an Old Testament law, or just choose to test God's rules, but you will pay for it. Even if you disagree with the law of gravity, God put it in place, and messing with it may end in dire results.

God's plan for eating is the same. God told Adam in Genesis 2:16, *"You are free to eat from any tree in the garden"* (except for the tree of the knowledge of good and evil, of course!), and after the flood, in Genesis 9:3, He said, *"Everything that lives and moves will be food for you."* Plants and animals live and move. Chemicals do not live and move. God gave us the plants and animals of the earth to eat, but much of what we are eating is chemicals. Our bodies are paying the price for our lack of obedience to God's Word. If we choose to eat differently than

God designed our bodies to eat, we need to be ready to live with the consequences. Paul puts it best in I Corinthians 10:31, *"So whatever you eat or drink or whatever you do, do it all for the glory of God."*

Even with this book as your guide to shortcuts toward better health, it will take more time to eat healthy than some of our favorite forms of cooking that involve opening a box and turning on the microwave. I now save my time by not making as many trips to the doctor's office and not needing to take naps because I feel tired. Contracting cancer changes your life. Doctors' visits become part of your daily routine. I'd rather spend time cutting and chopping fresh, organic fruits and vegetables than going to chemotherapy and radiation treatments. Ask your friends who have had cancer. Change your diet while you still have the chance.

Eating as recommended in this book keeps our bodies alkaline, a key to maintaining our health.

Eating well changes where you spend your money. Rather than twice-weekly trips to Starbucks costing $4 each, a soda and chips at the gas station convenience store for $10, $12 for family sodas at restaurants and miscellaneous junk food purchases, I choose to spend more money on fruits, vegetables and hormone-free meat. We feel better and know we are doing something good for ourselves.

My traditional medical doctors' bills are almost nonexistent. Unless someone at our house is injured, we hardly ever need to go to the traditional medical doctor. On occasion, we go to the chiropractic doctor for preventive maintenance. The biggest reason for bankruptcy in America is major health problems. I choose to spend my money on the positives of health food that will increase the energy and well-being of our family.

Are you overwhelmed? Don't worry. Don't do the whole *Shopper's Guide to Healthy Living* process at once. It has taken our family many years to get to Phase V, and we often regress (like on holidays or birthdays) and go back and "cheat." That's okay. We are still much healthier than before we started. When we cheat for any length of time, like vacations or holidays, we usually notice that one or more family members get sick and we are again motivated to eat better and live well.

If it seems too overwhelming, just go back and reread Phase I. Implement that phase for several months. When Phase I seems simple to you, the changes have become second nature, and you are feeling better, read Phase II and implement that section. Do the same with each phase. After you have experimented with different brands of products, start purchasing them in bulk. Eating and living healthy really can be simple; we just have to relearn how to do it in today's society. You can do it and it is worth it!

There are poisons all around us, but we do not need to get paranoid or worried. We just need to be aware of potential poisons in our environment, eliminate those we can, keep the ones we are unwilling to give up, and live with the ones we cannot control. At least then our bodies will have a fighting chance, and we can control our own health in today's exciting world.

God bless you and your family on your quest to healthier living!

Tear-out Shopping Lists

Tear out these lists and take them shopping with you. I have included a second list to be left in the book for future reference.

--- ✂

PHASE I

Purchase:
Extra virgin olive oil/walnut oil
Free-range eggs w/omega 3's
Organic butter
Organic fruits and vegetables
Ezekiel Sprouted Grain breads/Great Harvest/
      Rudy's Organic bread
POM juice
Flax seed
Hormone-free meats/chicken
Natural chips
Organic cookies and crackers
All natural ice cream

Eliminate:
Partially hydrogenated oils
High fructose corn syrup
Vegetable oils
Lard/Crisco/margarine
Non-organic fruits and vegetables
White bread
Clothes dryer sheets
Meat/chicken with hormones
Farm raised fish
National brand chips
Non-organic cookies and crackers
Ice creams with high fructose corn syrup

-- ✂

PHASE II

Purchase:
Household water filter
Organic peanut butter
Clif and Luna Bars
Fresh-ground spelt flour
Organic deodorant and tampons
Organic milk and cheese
Wild, cold- water fish
Local raw honey
Organic cold cereals and granolas
Long-cooking, fresh-ground oatmeal
Organic shampoos, soaps and lotions
Organic coffee
Peppermint oil

Eliminate:
Plastic water bottles
Peanut butter with partially hydrogenated oil
Grocery store deodorant and tampons
Non-organic milk and cheese
Seafood without fins and scales
Honey that is not raw
Non organic cereals and granolas
Instant oatmeal
Non organic shampoos, soaps and lotions
Non-organic coffee/creamers
Pop/soda
NSAIDs (non steroidal anti-inflammatory pain relievers)
Food containing color dyes
Lotions containing sodium lauryl sulfate, propylene
glycol, color dyes

- -
- -

PHASE III

Purchase:
Goat's milk and cheese
Bread machine and/or grain mill
Pro-biotics
Maple syrup
Agave nectar
Organic lemons
Hormone/nitrate-free lunch meats
Organic condiments

Eliminate:
Cow's milk
Store-bought pancake syrup
Grocery store lunch meats/salami/pepperoni
Non-organic condiments
Bacon/pork products
Fast-food meals
Artificial sweeteners

PHASE IV

Purchase:
Almond milk
Raw nuts
More raw fruits and vegetables
Experiment with separating your foods
Remaining white flour/sugar in your diet
Herbal Teas
Organic onions and garlic
Aluminum-free baking powder
Organic package seasonings/condiments
Organic bug spray
Sea salt
Natural chewing gum

Eliminate:
Cooked/vacuum-sealed nuts
Potatoes and corn
Coffee
Baking powder/tortillas with aluminum
Non-organic seasonings/condiments
Bug spray with DEET
Table salt with aluminum
Chewing gum with aspartame
Aluminum foil

PHASE V

Purchase or begin:
Dry brush for lymph nodes
Looking for a doctor of chiropractic
Juice fast items (juicer)
Green drinks
Organic sunscreen/makeup/nail polishes
Organic candles
Phosphate and dye-free laundry/dish soap
Stainless steel pots/pans/spatulas
Glass jars
Supplements
Magic Cloth
Natural toothpaste

Eliminate:
Perfume
Non-organic sunscreen/makeup/nail polish
Petroleum-based candles/products
Soaps with phosphates/dyes
Non-stick pots/pans/spatulas
Plastic food-storage containers
Household chemicals
Grocery store toothpaste

Tear-out Shopping Lists

Extra copy for future reference.

PHASE I

Purchase:
Extra virgin olive oil/Walnut oil
Free-range eggs w/omega 3's
Organic butter
Organic fruits and vegetables
Ezekiel Sprouted Grain breads/Great Harvest/
         Rudy's Organic bread
POM juice
Flax seed
Hormone-free meats/chicken
Natural chips
Organic cookies and crackers
All natural ice cream

Eliminate:
Partially hydrogenated oils
High fructose corn syrup
Vegetable oils
Lard/Crisco/margarine
Non-organic fruits and vegetables
White bread
Sugary fruit juices
Clothes dryer sheets
Meat/chicken with hormones
Farm-raised fish
National brand chips
Non-organic cookies and crackers
Ice creams with high fructose corn syrup

PHASE II

Purchase:
Household water filter
Organic peanut butter
Clif and Luna Bars
Fresh-ground spelt flour
Organic deodorant and tampons
Organic milk and cheese
Wild, cold- water fish
Local raw honey
Organic cold cereals and granolas
Long-cooking, fresh-ground oatmeal
Organic shampoos, soaps and lotions
Organic coffee
Peppermint oil

Eliminate:
Plastic water bottles
Peanut butter with partially hydrogenated oil
Grocery store deodorant and tampons
Non-organic milk and cheese
Seafood without fins and scales
Honey that is not raw
Non organic cereals and granolas
Instant oatmeal
Non organic shampoos, soaps and lotions
Non-organic coffee/creamers
Pop/soda
NSAIDs (non steroidal anti-inflammatory pain relievers)

PHASE III

Purchase:
Goat's milk and cheese
Bread machine and/or grain mill
Pro-biotics
Maple syrup
Agave nectar
Organic lemons
Hormone/nitrate-free lunch meats
Organic condiments

Eliminate:
Cow's milk
Store-bought pancake syrup
Grocery store lunch meats/salami/pepperoni
Non-organic condiments
Bacon/pork products
Fast-food meals
Artificial sweeteners

PHASE IV

Purchase:
Almond milk
Raw nuts
More raw fruits and vegetables
Experiment with separating your foods
Remaining white flour/sugar in your diet
Herbal Teas
Organic onions and garlic
Aluminum-free baking powder
Organic package seasonings/condiments
Organic bug spray
Sea salt
Natural chewing gum

Eliminate:
Cooked/vacuum-sealed nuts
Potatoes and corn
Coffee
Baking powder/tortillas with aluminum
Non-organic seasonings/condiments
Bug spray with DEET
Table salt with aluminum
Chewing gum with aspartame
Aluminum foil

PHASE V

Purchase or begin:
Dry brush for lymph nodes
Looking for a doctor of chiropractic
Juice fast items (juicer)
Green drinks
Organic sunscreen/makeup/nail polishes
Organic candles
Phosphate and dye-free laundry/dish soap
Stainless steel pots/pans/spatulas
Glass jars
Supplements
Magic Cloth
Natural toothpaste

Eliminate:
Perfume
Non-organic sunscreen/makeup/nail polish
Petroleum-based candles/products
Soaps with phosphates/dyes
Non-stick pots/pans/spatulas
Plastic food-storage containers
Household chemicals
Grocery store toothpaste

Recipes for Healthy Living

Whole Grain Pancakes

Dry ingredients:
1½ cups ground spelt flour
1/8 cup ground flax seeds
3 t. aluminum-free baking powder
1 t. sea salt

Wet ingredients:
3 eggs
3 T olive oil or walnut oil
1 t. pure vanilla
1 cup goat or almond milk
Stir dry ingredients together. Combine wet ingredients in a separate bowl. Add to dry ingredients. Bake on a lightly oiled stove top griddle.

Delicious Waffles

Dry ingredients:
2 ½ - 3 cups ground spelt flour
1/8 cup ground flax seeds
1 t. sea salt
3 t. baking powder

Wet ingredients:
3 beaten eggs
2 cups goat's milk or almond milk
2 T. olive oil or walnut oil
1 t. pure vanilla
1. T. raw honey

Stir dry ingredients together. In separate bowl, combine wet ingredients. Add to dry ingredients. Bake on waffle maker, lightly greased with olive oil

Whole Grain Spelt Bread
By Donna Poelstra

9 cups whole grain spelt flour—ground in mill to make 12 cups ground flour
½ cup olive oil or walnut oil
½ cup honey
3 T. SAF instant yeast
2 T. Real sea salt
¼ cup ground flax seed
1 T. dough enhancer—optional
5 cups warm water

Mix ingredients in a Bosch bread machine. Put into 4 greased stainless steel loaf pans. Bake at 350° for 30 minutes.

• *To order Donna's cookbooks, go to TasteofLifeStores.com*

Healthy Oatmeal Cookies

Dry ingredients:
3 ½-4 cups ground whole grain flour
3 cups ground oats
1 t. baking soda
1 cup raisins
1 t. baking powder
½ cup chopped walnuts
1 t. salt
1 t. cinnamon
1 t. nutmeg
1 t. ginger

Wet ingredients:
1 cup melted butter
1 cup raw honey
3 eggs
½ cup goat's milk or almond milk
¾ t. vanilla

Combine first seven dry ingredients in a large bowl. In a separate bowl, combine the wet ingredients in mixer, cream for eight minutes. Add last three dry ingredients to other dry ingredients, combine. Stir wet ingredients into the dry mix, just until combined.

Drop onto greased cookie sheet, press down with the bottom of a greased glass. Bake at 350° for nine minutes.

Oatmeal Muffins
By Joan Decker and Susan Sullivan

Dry ingredients:
2 cups ground oat groats or oat meal
1¼ cups ground spelt flour
¼ cup ground flax seed
1 t. cinnamon
1 t. baking powder
½ t. baking soda
½ t. sea salt

Wet ingredients;
1 cup goat's milk or almond milk
½ cup raw honey
¼ cup olive oil or walnut oil
2 beaten eggs
1 cup blueberries

Combine dry ingredients and set aside. Combine first four wet ingredients, add to the dry ingredients. Mix just until moist. Add blueberries. Place in greased muffin pans 2/3 full. Bake at 425° for 18-25 minutes.

Whole Grain Bread Crumbs
By Kathy Weiler

Use leftover bread crusts and heels that have been stored in a freezer bag. Place them in a single layer on a cookie sheet. Bake at 350° for 10-15 minutes, or until toasty. Bread should be hard.

Grind 2-4 pieces of toast at a time in a blender, until all are crumbly. Place bread crumbs in a large bowl and spice to taste.

Suggested spices for 4 cups bread crumbs:
4 T. garlic salt
3 T. oregano
3 T. onion salt
3 T. seasoned salt

Whole Grain Croutons
By Kathy Weiler

Cut old pieces of whole grain bread into 1-inch squares. Sprinkle with olive oil, oregano, thyme, parsley, garlic and other desired herbs. Place on greased cookie sheet, in one layer.

Bake at 350° for 20-30 minutes, until golden brown.

Teriyaki Salmon
By Matt Loidolt

Grease baking dish with olive oil to prevent sticking. Place slab of salmon scale side down in dish.

Top with: garlic powder
              Seasoned salt
              Pepper
              Organic teriyaki sauce
              Dot with butter

Bake at 350° for 15-20 minutes, depending on thickness of the salmon.

Garlic Halibut
By Matt Loidolt

Grease baking dish with olive oil to prevent sticking. Place halibut scale side down in dish.

Top with: Garlic salt
              Sea salt
              Pepper
              Dot with butter

Bake at 350° for 20-25 minutes.

Healthy (and still good-tasting) Brown Bag Lunch Sample

Hormone-free turkey meat on homemade or natural bread or organic peanut or almond butter on homemade or natural bread
fresh cut fruit or vegetables—2 or 3 different kinds
organic nuts
organic chips if needed

RO water
Clif or Luna bar for dessert

This lunch is incredibly healthy and still tastes good. It may take awhile for your kids to get used to it. You may want to phase it in. It still does not address the Raw Food Detox Diet's separation of food types. Therefore, I suggest to my children that they eat their fruit at snack time.

Homemade Pancake Syrup

1 cup boiling water
2 cups pure cane juice or white sugar
½ t. imitation maple flavoring

Pour 1 cup boiling water over 2 cups sugar, stir. Add maple flavor and stir again. Makes 2 ½ cups.

Fresh Oatmeal
By Donna Poelstra

Grind 1 cup oat groats.

Boil 2 cups water in saucepan. Add 1 cup oat groats. Cook 20 minutes on low heat, stirring often.

Serve hot with butter, honey and bananas, if desired.

Resources

Bread making machines and lessons

Taste of Life
(719) 487-2858
Donna@TasteofLifeStores.com

Blood typing kits

Eldon Biologicals A/S
D/K-2820, Gentofte, Denmark
Eldoncard@Eldoncard.com

Craigmedical.com

Bulk ordering

Back to the Basics Natural Foods
(719) 532-0553

Chiropractors

Colorado Health and Wellness
www.Colorado Health and Wellness.com
(719) 576-2225

Free Range Meat

Searle Ranch
(719) 481-3735

Premium Meats
(866) 71-MEATS
www.prairienaturalmeats.com

Juicers

Champion Juicer
622 E. Hwy 12
Lodi, CA 95240
(209) 369-2154
www.Championjuicer.com

Omega Juicer
Omega Products, Inc.
Harrisburg, PA 17111-4523
(717) 561-1105

Vita Mix
www.vitamix.com

Magic Cloths

www.magiccloth.com

Makeup

Arbonne
Representative Leiph McHugh
hadleyray@msn.com
(719) 481-5630

Naturopathics
Bella Vi
(719) 487-3123

Organic food markets and organic personal chefs

Homemade Goodness
(719) 481-3398
Tonja Gibson

Isagenix
www.healthystart09.isagenix.com

Sprouts

Sun Flower Market

Taste of Life
(719) 487-2858
Donna@TasteofLifeStores.com

The Wedge

Trader Joe's

Vitamin Cottage

Vitamin Shoppe

Whole Foods

Wild Oats

Water filtering systems

Affordable Water Service
(719) 548-0313

Product Favorites

One of the most expensive things about eating and living healthier is purchasing all the products you want to try in order to find one or two brands that your family will like. Therefore, I have done this work for you. I have purchased and sampled many products and have found many good replacements for the old SAD diet items. Here is a list of some of the products my family has enjoyed as "different but still good," or at least decided are "not disgusting." There are many other good products on the market; these have just become our personal new favorites.

Most of these products can be purchased at your local health food store. If not, I have included the Web site or phone number.

I do not own the companies that make these products. I just want to save you time and money by giving you a place to start looking for food and personal products that are "different, but still good."

Food Products:

Apple Cider Vinegar—Bragg's Raw Unfiltered Organic

Bars
       Artisto Body and Mind

Clif—Chocolate Brownie/Cookies and Cream
Kashi—GOLEAN Peanut Butter & Chocolate/
        Cookies & Cream/Chocolate Malted Milk
Luna—Smores/Chai Tea/Mint & Chocolate
Supreme Protein
Yotta Bar

Butter/Cheese

Alta Dena
Earth Balance
Horizon Organic
Karoun Dairies
Organic Earth Balance Butter Spread
Organic Valley
Willow River
Woodstock Farms

Cereals

Barbara's Whole Oat Cereal Apple Cinnamon
        Toasted O's
Barbara's Bakery Puffins—cinnamon
Barbara's Shredded Wheat
Cascadian Farms Cinnamon Raisin Granola
Cascadian Farms Multi Grain /
        Vanilla Almond Crunch Granola
Cascadian Farms Oats and Honey Granola
Cascadian Farms Organic Purely O's
Cascadian Farms Raisin Bran
Kashi GOLEAN Crunch
Kashi Heart to Heart
Mountain Madness Granola

Chips, etc.

Boulder Canyon Hickory BBQ Potato Chips
Frontera Stone Ground

Garden of Eatin Yellow Chips
Guiltless Gourmet Chili Lime/Chili Verde/Blue Chips
Have' A Corn Chips
Kettle Tortilla Chips—Organic
Little Bear Snack Foods Original Baked Cheddar Puffs
Lundberg Baked Rice Twists
Mexi Snax Sesame/ Salted Original/Nacho
Natural Tostitos/Cheetos/Cheese Chips
Newman's Own Pretzels – any type
Pirate Booty Corn/Smart Puffs
Purity Foods Spelt Pretzels
Que Pasa Organic White Corn Tortilla Chips/Yellow
    Corn Tortilla Chips
Regenie's Chips

Crackers/Cookies

Alvarado St Bakery Goods
Annie's Cheddar Bunnies
Back to Nature Crispy Wheats baked snack crackers
Betty Lou's
Blue Diamond Nut Thins
Dessert Bowls
Ice Box Bakery
Kashi TLC or any kind
Late July Organic—any type
Midel Vanilla/ Ginger Snaps
My Family Farm Cheddar Cheese
Newman's Own Newman O's/Champion Chip/
    Fig Newton's
Newman's Own Chocolate Alphabet Cookies/
    Ginger O's
Our Family Farm—any type

Drinks

Cherrish
Hansen's Natural
Health and Energy Water
Izze Sparkling Soda
MIX Protein & Antioxidant Drink
POM Wonderful Pomegranate Blueberry 100 Percent
        Juice
Recharge Thirst Quenchers
Sparka Natural Drink
Vitamin Water

Frozen Snacks
Alexia Snacks Ham & Cheese Stuffed Sandwiches
Amy's Cheese Lasagna/Enchilada/Mac & Cheese
Amy's Spinach Pizza-in-a-Pocket Sandwich/Pizza
Amy's Bowls Ravioli/Vegetable Pot Pie
Full Tank
Hallelujah Chicken
Health is Wealth Spinach Munchees
Health is Wealth Spring Rolls
Kim & Scott's Gourmet Pretzels
Michael Angelo's Lasgne
Mom Made

Gum
XyliChew

Ketchup
Heinz Organic Tomato Ketchup
Muir Glen Organic Tomato Ketchup
Woodstock Farms

Kitchenware
Nutriware by Aroma
www.mynutriware.com

Milk

    Meyenberger Goat Milk
    Almond Breeze—Vanilla and Chocolate

Packaged Seasoning Mixes/Sauces

    Simply Organic Alfredo/Sweet Basil/Pesto/Southwest
        Taco/Fajita
    Muir Glen Organic Pizza Sauce
    Evan's Front Range Salsa

Pasta

    Vita Spelt—any style
    Pasta Joy Brown Rice Pasta
    Road's End Organics

Peanut Butter

    Maranatha Creamy Peanut Butter

Salad Dressing

    Annie's Cowgirl Ranch Dressing
    Cardini's Caesar Dressing
    Cindy's Kitchen Chipotle Ranch Dressing
    Cindy's Kitchen Wild Maine Blueberry Antioxidant
        Dressing

Salt

    REAL Sea Salt
    Celtic Salt

Yogurt

    Horizon—all flavors
    Stonyfield—all flavors

Teas

Yogi Tea Echinacea Immune Support
Raspberry Ginger
Peppermint
Ginger
Choice Organic Teas—Chamomile Herb Teas

More Product Favorites—Personal Products:

Cleaners
> Earth Friendly Products
> Seventh Generation Products
> Unico Wipex Natural Wipes

Deodorant
> Alba
> Kiss My Face
> Nature's Gate Organics
> Chamomile and Lemon Verbena

Eye Cream
> Alba moisture cream
> L'uvalla
> Naturapathica

Fabric Softener
> Seventh Generation

Hair Spray
> Jason Thin-to-Thick
> Giovanni – LA Hold

Insect Repellent
> All Terrain Herbal Armor Spray insect repellent

Lip Balm
> Burt's Bees

Lotions
> Alba Cocoa Butter

ABRA Detox skin
Burt's Bees Milk and Honey Body Lotion
Ecco Bella
Kiss My Face
Nature's Finest Flax.com 1-619-838-7317
Pure and Basic Fuji Apple Berry

Makeup

Arbonne
Jane Eridal
L'uvalla
Naturopathics
Sinclair & Vitentine

Shampoo/Conditioner

Alba Volumizing
Avalon Organics
EO
Jason Thin-to-Thick
Mill Creek Henna

Soaps

Aspen Soap Company (719) 232-4837
Avalon Organics
Clearly Natural
EO
JASON
Kiss My Face
Nature's Gate
River Soap Company
Sappo Hill

Skin/Hand

JASON Lavender Satin Soap for Face and Hands
South of France

Soap for Clothes
Seventh Generation

Soap for Dishes
Earth Friendly Products High Performance Wave Auto Dishwasher
Ecover Ecological Dishwashing Liquid

Sunscreen

Alba Botanica SUN Organic

Toothpaste

Natural Whitening Gel Dental Therapy
Nature's Gate Crème De Mint
Nature's Gate Herbal Crème Natural Toothpaste
Nature's Gate Cool Mint Gel Natural Toothpaste
Nature's Gate Dental Therapy Whitening Gel
For kids: Tom's of Maine Natural Care Silly Strawberry

The "Forbidden List"

These ingredients need to be on our "do not eat" list. Use this list to check the ingredients of products you are purchasing. If the product contains any of these ingredients, find a healthy substitute.

Do not purchase food products that contain:

> Aluminum
> Aspartame
> Bleach
> Color dyes
> Cottonseed oil
> High fructose corn syrup
> MSG (Monosodium Glutamate), which also doubles as:
>> autolyzed yeast
>> calcium caseinate
>> hydrolyzed oat flour
>> hydrolyzed plant protein
>> hydrolyzed protein
>> hydrolyzed vegetable protein
>> plant protein extract
>> sodium caseinate
>> textured protein
>> yeast extract
>> natural and artificial flavorings
> Nitrates
> Nitrites

Partially hydrogenated oils
White sugar, which also doubles as:
      concentrated grape juice
      fructose
      glucose
      sucrose
      sucralose (anything that rhymes with "gross"!)

Do not purchase personal care products that contain:

    Bleach
    Chlorine
    Color dyes
    EDTA
    Formaldehyde
    PABAs (para-aminobenzoic acids)
    Parabens
    Phosphates
    Propylene glycol
    Sodium lauryl sulfate

Kathy can be contacted for:

Group Seminars – private companies
large/small groups
schools
from one hour to all day
Family Pantry Makeovers
Personal Consulting

To get her weekly emails, order a book
or request the above services, go to
www.ShoppersGuidetoHealthyLiving.com
click on contact me or
email kloidolt@hotmail.com.

Notes

(Endnotes)

1   "Obesity Threatens to Cut U.S. Life Expectancy, New Analysis Suggests", U.S. Department of Health and Human Services, March 16, 2005

2   Reese Dubin, *Miracle Food Cures from the Bible*, Prentice Hall Press, 1999, pgs 229-230, 233-235, 242, 244-245

3   United States at Large 59th Congress, Session 1, 3915, 768-772

4   http://www.fda.review.org/history.shtmlthird

5   http:/www.westonaprice.org/motherlinda/cornsyrup.html

6   Dr. Larraine Day DVD, "Cancer Doesn't Scare Me Anymore", produced by Rockford Press, 2002

7   Veggie Tale Videos produced by Big Idea Productions, 1995

8   Konrad Kail, N.D. and Bobbi Lawrence, with Burton Goldberg, *Allergy Free*, Alternative Medicine.com, Inc., CA, 2000

9   Karen Klonsky, "The Organic Foods Production Act: How Will Implementation Change the Face of California's Organic Agriculture?", Department of Agriculture and Resource Economics, 2003

10 Michael Murray, N.D. and Joseph Pizzoro, N.D., *Encyclopedia of*

Natural Medicine, Three Rivers Press, NY, 1997, pg 95

11   Eric Schlosser, *Fast Food Nation, Harper Perennial,* Harper Perennial, NY, 2004, pgs 272-275_

12   "Shop Smart", Consumer Reports, February 2006, pg14

13   http://www.natural ingredient.org/naturalingredient.html

14   "The Poisoning of Our Foods", Professor Rozalind A Gruben, Courtesy of Healthful Living International

15   Andrew Weil. *Eight Weeks to Optimum Health,* Random House Publishing Group, NY, 1997, pg 84-85

16   "Shop Smart", Consumer Reports, February 2006, pg14

17   "The Poisoning of Our Foods", Professor Rozalind A Gruben, Courtesy of Healthful Living International

18   www.whfoods.com/genpage.php?tname=foodspice&dbid=143-32K

19   http://www.pacificbakery.com/spelt/htm

20   Reese Dubin. *Miracle Food Cures from the Bible*, Prentice Hall Press, 1999, pgs 12-13

21   Annybelle Foundation Advanced Health Plan Website 2001-2005

22   Michael Murray, N.D. and Joseph Pizzorno, N.D. *Encyclopedia of Natural Medicine*, Three Rivers Press, pg 53

23   http://sweetpoison.com/aboutsweetpoison.html

24   Michael Murray, N.D. and Joseph Pizzorno, N.D. *Encyclopedia of Natural Medicine*, Three Rivers Press, pgs 274-277

25   http://www.whfoods.com/genpage.php?tname=foodspice&dbid=143

26 http://www.whfoods.com/genpage.php?tname=foodspice&dbi
    d=143

27 Kevin Trudeau, *Natural Cures They Don't Want You to Know*,
    Alliance Publishing Group, Inc.,2004, pgs 137-138

28 Dr. Bill Swallow, Nitrates and Nitrites: Dietary Exposure and Risks
    Assessments, Institute of Environmental Science and Research
    Limited, New Zealand, FW0392, pg 8

29 http://sweetpoison.com/aboutsweetpoison.html

30 http://www.rense.com/general52/msg.tml

31 Natalie Rose, The Raw Food Detox Diet, Regan Books, 2005

32 Reese Dubin. *Miracle Food Cures from the Bible*, Prentice Hall
    Press, 1999, pg 332

33 Dr. Peter J.D'Adamo, *Eat Right For Your Blood Type*, G.P. Putnam's
    Sons Publishing, NY 1996

34 Cheryl Townsend, *Cleansing Made Simple*, LFH Publishing, CO,
    2001

35 David Fraum. *Health Quarters Monthly*, December 2005 issue

36 *"Neurotoxins: At Home and the Workplace"*, Report by the Com-
    mittee on Science and Technology, U.S. House of Representa-
    tives, Sept 16, 1986 (Report 99-827)